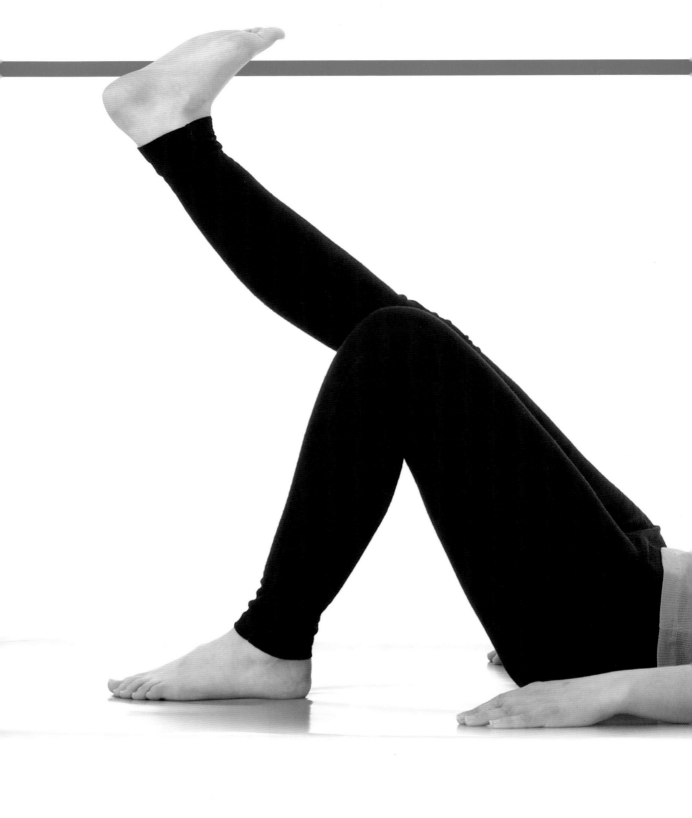

PILATES
FOR EQUESTRIANS

Achieve the winning edge
with increased
core stability

LIZA RANDALL

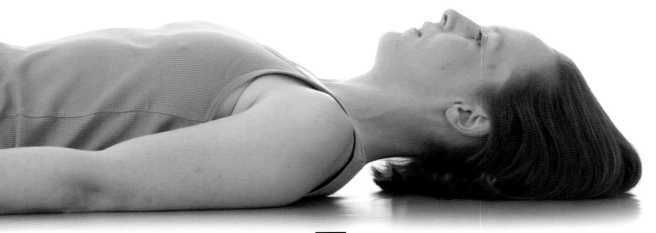

Kenilworth Press

First published in the UK in 2010
by Kenilworth Press, an imprint of Quiller Publishing Ltd

British Library Cataloguing-in-Publication Data
A catalogue record for this book
is available from the British Library

ISBN 978 1 905693 34 4

Studio photography by Simon Lusty; mounted and other outdoor photographs
by the author and Karl Randall.

Line illustrations and cartoons by Dianne Breeze.

Book and cover design by Sharyn Troughton.

Printed in China

Kenilworth Press
An imprint of Quiller Publishing Ltd
Wykey House, Wykey, Shrewsbury, SY4 1JA
Tel: 01939 261616 Fax: 01939 261606
E-mail: info@quillerbooks.com
Website: www.kenilworthpress.co.uk

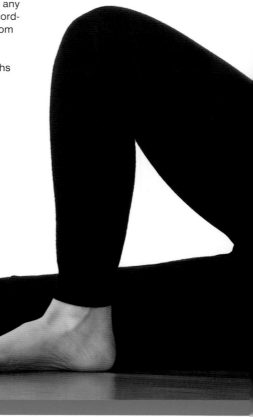

Contents

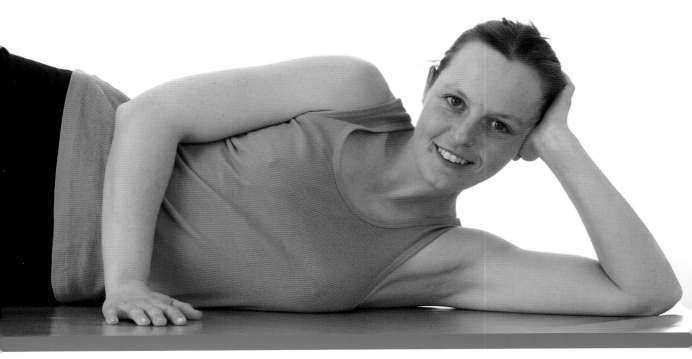

Exercises From Front-lying or Prone

Exercises From Four-point Kneeling

Exercises From Side-lying

Acknowledgements

A huge thank-you to my family for supporting me in this endeavour; a special thanks to my mum, Moira, for helping to look after my premature baby Tom, who unexpectedly arrived mid-book!

Thank you to patient photographer Simon Lusty for the studio photography. A hundred thanks go to my horsy friends and clients for taking part in the photo-shoots. I wanted this book to reflect a myriad of gorgeous, real life, body shapes, sizes and ages; not look like a glossy photo-shoot of long-legged beauties with perfect postures. All the riders featured take weekly classes and benefit from the mind-body approach that is Body Control Pilates. A special thanks to professional advanced event rider, Deborah Fielding, a five-foot dynamo whose lovely grace has been captured in the pages of this book; her movement and strength have been enhanced and improved by Pilates. Then to the two Janets for being guinea pigs with their lovely mounts, Valdi and Oscar.

Thank you also for the blessing of Pilates guru Lynne Robinson and Body Control Pilates® Association (see www.bodycontrol.co.uk to look up details of your local Pilates instructor).

Lastly, thank you to Kate Fernyhough, physiotherapist extraordinaire, for wading through copy and for introducing me in the first place to the life-changing rehabilitating, exhilarating and body conditioning method that is Pilates.

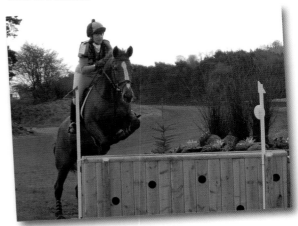

Foreword

As riders, we take great care of our horses – with vets, equine physios, farriers and other specialists and trainers on hand. They spring into action at a moment's notice if we think there is anything wrong, or if we are not achieving our riding goals. But what about the rider's physical and psychological needs? How often have you called the physiotherapist or osteopath to look at a nagging ache, or taken time out to do something for yourself? You can probably count the times on one hand!

More and more, athletes are realising the benefits from improved core stability, which can be achieved through Pilates. Olympic skiers, rowers, rugby players, triathletes and jockeys have all tried it and triumphed, and so include it into their conditioning programme. This is not just to improve their performance on the day, but also to help prevent injury by targeting the deep postural muscles that balance their body. Regular riders now have the opportunity to add a Pilates workout to their daily routine and enjoy its benefits for life. Once you have the Pilates principles and basic exercises off pat, you'll be amazed at how much better you will feel overall; you'll begin to walk tall and hold yourself with more presence, benefiting from increased strength from the inside out.

Pilates is a simple concept which centres on core stability. And for riders it makes sense, as the same principle applies to the horse. To give a horse lift and strength so that he can engage his hocks and shoulders correctly, his powerhouse, or abdominal muscles must be engaged and then he can become round and 'through' and soft in the back. A hollow horse is simply not using his muscles correctly – the same comment can be applied to a person.

The best thing about Pilates is that it is for everyone – regardless of your age, physical ability or size. Using this programme, you can pick and choose what exercises to do as they are all colour-flagged in five stages, with orange your beginner exercises, through to pink, yellow, green and red.

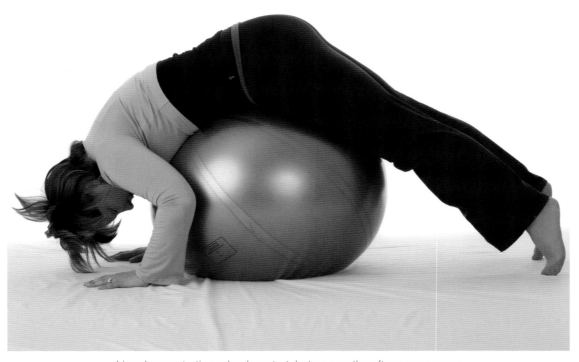

Liza demonstrating a lumbar stretch, two months after a caesarean.

About the Author

I first came to Pilates purely by accident – literally. I came a cropper showjumping in an indoor school when trying to jump-off faster than everyone else!

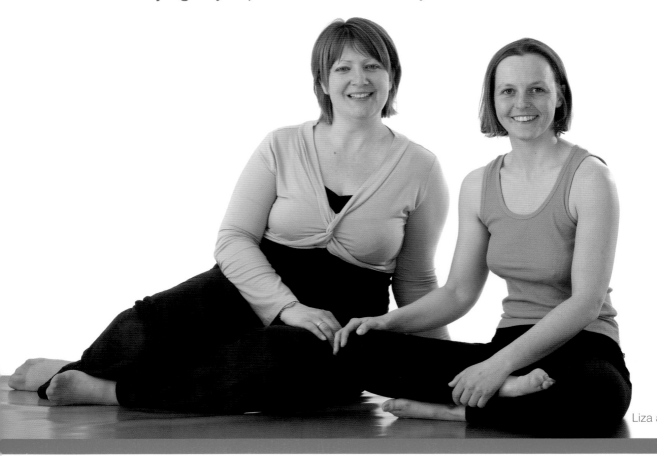

Liza and D

After being shipped off to Shrewsbury hospital on a spinal board, I knew I had done a bit of damage. I remember pleading with the doctors, saying I had to get to an appointment the next day in the West Country so I would be grateful if they could give me some painkillers and I would be on my way – sadly, that was not to be. I had burst several vertebrae in my lumbar spine, an unstable injury, so I had to remain motionless on my back until a place came up at a specialist unit. Three weeks later I got the call and was transferred for expert treatment at the wonderful Oswestry Orthopaedic.

So, a few months down the line and a pioneering metal body cage later, I was learning how to sit up, stand and take a few steps. Hydrotherapy, physiotherapy and then Pilates followed – I was one of the lucky ones to get back up on my feet.

My story is not dissimilar from that of many people who ride – backs and necks are at the root of many problems, purely because the spine is the longest 'string' of bones in the body, it means these areas are vulnerable to injury. And not as a result of falling, but just as easily through incorrect posture, poor body awareness or incorrect muscle patterning.

Liza and Pilates

Liza was trained by Lynne Robinson and her highly skilled Pilates teacher-trainers at the London Body Control Pilates Association (BCPA). She was then mentored by chartered physiotherapist and Pilates teacher Kate Fernyhough in Staffordshire – an inspirational teacher who first introduced Liza to Pilates following her accident. Liza then went on to teach at Pilates studios in London, Warwickshire, Cheshire and Northamptonshire and took her final exams to achieve her full qualifications as a Level 3 Pilates coach with the BCPA. With an interest in coaching sportsmen and women, particularly equestrians, Liza founded Panacea Pilates and now teaches Pilates to professional and amateur riders alike in Worcestershire and Gloucestershire, as well as eventing her own horses in her spare time.

Liza and Rose

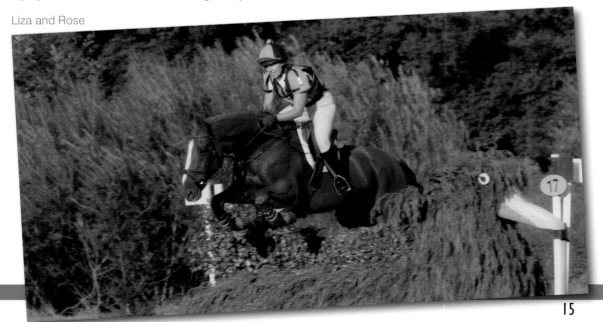

Origins of Pilates

From pop stars to movie stars, it seems every celebrity has a tale to tell about the benefits of Pilates. But where did it come from? Pilates is not a new 'fad'. Its origins are in the 1880s with its founder, Joseph Pilates. Joseph was born in Germany, and was a rather sickly boy who suffered with repeated illnesses whilst growing up. It was from these beginnings that he became obsessed with the perfect body and exercising in the outdoors. He strove to improve his own body through a variety of exercises, including martial arts.

Joseph moved to England in 1912, where he worked as a self-defence instructor to the detectives at Scotland Yard. When the First World War broke out, Joseph was interned with other German nationals in the UK. In his camp, he trained other internees and spent a lot of his time in the infirmary, helping bedridden patients to regain muscle function by training them to work against resistance to help build the body, by rigging up a variety of springs to hospital beds. These ideas later became used in the building of his Pilates exercise machines.

When a flu epidemic struck England in 1918, none of Joseph's trainees died, which he claimed was a testament to the success of his method of mind-body exercise.

After the war, Joseph returned to Germany, where he took his exercises to the dance community who benefited from the extra strength it gave them when added to their repertoire, and he was soon in great demand. News of his methods spread, but when he was asked by the German government to train the German army in his fitness techniques, he decided to quit Germany for good and emigrated to America in 1926. It was on the boat over to the USA that Joseph met his wife-to-be, Clara. They made New York their home and set up a fitness studio in a building they shared with the New York City Ballet.

By the 1960s, the Pilates method was well-known and practised by many dancers, and its popularity had spread throughout the United States.

Joseph continued to teach at his New York Studio until he died, aged 87, in 1967. Many people had passed through his studio and benefited from his teachings and went on to open their own studios. Pilates soon became the preferred exercise method of the Hollywood stars in the 1970s and its popularity continues today.

So why, you say, is Pilates – a method taught to dancers – of use to horse riders? It is because there are many parallels with both athletes. As a rider, you need to be able to control your horse, a powerful but sensitive animal, with just a twitch of a muscle here or a shift in weight there. A rider needs to be strong from the inside out, as does a dancer, with the ability to engage deep postural muscles for ultimate grace and flexibility in the dressage, stability and power in showjumping and quick reflexes, strength and endurance for successful cross-country riding. We'll explore these issues in more detail in the next chapter.

PART ONE

PILATES PRINCIPLES AND BASIC
CONSIDERATIONS

Why Riders Should do Pilates

W e've just seen some core reasons why; now, let's examine the issue in more detail. Apart from the obvious physical benefits such as increased tone, a longer, leaner body, more flexibility and a better sense of awareness in the saddle, Pilates relaxes the body and mind and encourages the rider to breathe for maximum efficiency.

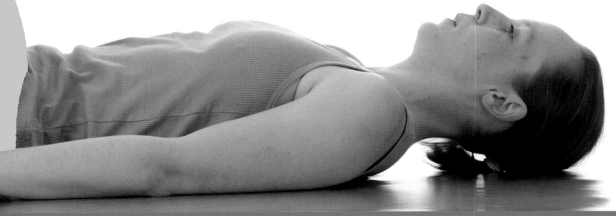

This breathing technique can be transferred to many situations the rider may face – whether it is going out for a hack on a fresh horse, preparation for riding down the centre line in a dressage test, or for when waiting in the start box about to go off across country. Pilates breathing allows a rider to centre themselves and see the whole picture – how to successfully tackle the task ahead – rather than just glimpsing pieces of the jigsaw, which is usually what happens when fear takes over.

A more natural, efficient posture is a lovely side-effect of Pilates as muscles are realigned. Because Pilates is a full-body workout, time is given to exercises in extension, so those improvements are transferred to when sitting in the saddle, with shoulders naturally realigned and shoulder-blades gently drawn down the back, abdominals lifted and tailbone under.

Pilates concentrates on using the smaller, inner stabilising muscles of the body rather than the major moving muscles, which are often overused. It has been found that riders can develop more 'feel' once they have discovered Pilates, as they are able to isolate, target and use these various muscles more discreetly and on command.

Riders who practise Pilates have often said that, even after just a few sessions, their body awareness improves and therefore so does their riding. For example Point and Flex and Ankle Circles (page 80) isolate and exercise the feet and ankle joints, achieving control of movement, so that once in the saddle a rider can move their foot slightly, sending a subtle command to the horse. Likewise, a gentle squeeze on the rein by the ring finger can ask a horse to half-halt. Body awareness and the control of your extremities can be fine-tuned so that you can gauge just how much body movement you need to use, until it can be so refined that control is achieved in a flowing and quiet way.

A rider needs the ability to flex and move the pelvis freely to absorb the horse's movement. Difficulties in this area can be identified by an excessive nod of the head when in the dressage arena; another telltale sign is uncontrollable leg movement when showjumping. A rider who can absorb the horse's movement without mirroring that movement in their own extremities, will ride with a much better seat – and you will see that the horse literally springs off the floor, as his own movement is not being blocked or stifled by his rider.

Once a rider understands the need to be stable through their pelvis, complex dressage movements with the horse become much easier – see Waist Twist (page 189). The ability to open the hip and lengthen the leg is essential for many riding movements, including most dressage exercises from leg-yield to canter changes. A showjumper needs strong gluteus medius muscles (see page 30) to change direction in the air around a twisty course and an eventer needs open hips for all phases and to stabilise them whilst riding across country in a two-point seat – see Oyster (page 142) and Leg Circles (page 88).

For example, a common mistake when riding shoulder-in is that the rider collapses through their inside waist and falls over to the inside as they try to create the bend. It is important when riding the movement to remain seated centrally in the saddle and allow the aiding leg to move instead. Another example is when performing travers. By learning to isolate and control the pelvis independently of both the upper and lower body, a rider is able to keep the pelvis centrally in the saddle, with hips facing forward, whilst turning the upper body – see Thread the Needle (page 132). A common mistake is to turn both shoulders and hips.

Depending on which discipline(s) they compete in, riders can develop various imbalances. For example, the thigh muscles can overdevelop, which then disadvantages the rider in the dressage phase. A common complaint of event riders is stiffness in the lower back and thighs, as a consequence of riding in the cross-country position. Pilates exercises to release the spine sequentially, such as Spine Curls (page 48) and Roll Down (page 61), practised in two different planes of movement, are highly beneficial to the rider. Eventers can also suffer from tight hamstrings, so stretches like the Hamstring Stretch (page 96) can be done in the lorry park before the cross-country phase. This is why Pilates, instead of pure strength work, is better for the rider as it creates suppleness and softness, rather than over-big muscles! Essentially all riders, no matter what the discipline, need the ability to be strong and firm one second, then loose and relaxed the next.

Lifting the ribs is another skill learnt in Pilates. A lifted (not flared) ribcage in a rider is like an elevated ribcage in a horse. Movements like passage, extended trot and a bouncy canter – which is essential for a showjumping combination or a rail/ditch/rail on the cross-country course become so much easier. Useful exercises for this are Ribcage Closure (page 94) or Studio Stretch (page 154).

By becoming more stable in the saddle, balance is improved. This is not only important for the dressage rider, but vital for jumping. Staying in harmony and focus over a difficult fence and being able to centre yourself, could mean the difference between staying with your horse or parting company if he makes an awkward jump!

Whatever discipline you enjoy with your horse, and whatever level you are at, whether riding is your weekend passion or your career, Pilates will give you added confidence in the saddle. If you compete, Pilates can offer you a winning edge.

And let's explode a myth right here – exercises involving the use of the pelvic floor muscles are not just for women! The Pilates method of 'contrology' was originally designed to get men injured in the war quickly back on their feet, and for those crippled with arthritis. Joseph Pilates focused on balance, strength, correcting muscle imbalances, improving co-ordination, posture and flexibility; all things he identified as being problems in 'modern' life.

Feel the benefits!

- Improved flexibility, co-ordination, balance, joint mobility
- Longer, leaner body with improved tone
- Improved posture
- Stress relief
- Improved vital organ function
- Boosted immune system
- Look and feel younger
- Respite from back pain

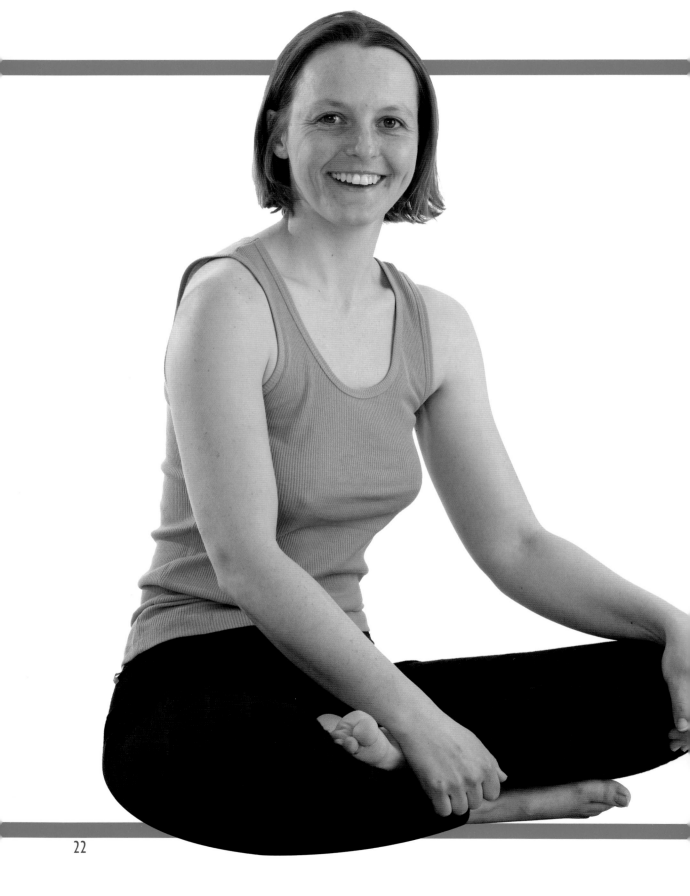

The Pilates Principles for Riders

When it comes to horses, we have the scales of training which are our basic ideals and foundations upon which riding is based – Pilates is the same. Whatever method of Pilates you choose to practise, you will come across similar principles. The main ones applicable to riders are outlined in the next three pages. If you find an exercise difficult, come down a level and re-examine the main principles, just as you would revisit the scales of training when learning a new movement with your horse.

Centring

Think of your internal deep muscles as your centre, like an apple core, which starts in the centre of your head, and passes down your neck into your upper and lower back, trunk and ribcage, ending in your pelvis. This is where your core stabilising muscles can be found. Core stability is essential for your posture and is your 'strength from within'. If you want to compare this term with your horse, think engagement. Your horse, if not engaged, is hollow. Not only is this an ugly sight, but he is not going to improve his way of going as he will not move efficiently or use his muscles to give him lift and presence – the same is true for people. Once you have engaged these muscles, you immediately protect your back from injury and strain when you exercise or move around in everyday activity.

The amount of centring needed to perform an exercise is important – you don't want to over-recruit the muscles as this can lead to bracing and tension, neither do you want to under-engage them as this will compromise your stability and leave yourself open to strain or injury if you are about to perform one of the more complex Pilates movements. Think of centring or core stability as you would your leg aid when riding. You need enough leg for the horse to move forward: too much and you shoot off balance as you brace and tense to get back in control; too little and it is like trotting through concrete with little or no lift or impulsion.

Breathing

Even though we do this every second of every day, there is breathing and there is breathing! If you have ever hot-footed it across the yard to catch an errant horse who has pulled back on his lead-rope and is heading for the open road, you will find that your breathing is rapid and shallow, and is concentrated in your shoulders and upper neck – this is your fear or flight reflex cutting in. This is a different type of breathing from what you would use when you are cantering across country, where you pace yourself for maximum efficiency – this breathing will be more concentrated in your centre and you will rhythmically draw in breaths of air.

In Pilates you need to breathe wide and deep into the sides of your ribcage. This is called thoracic or lateral breathing. To feel this, place your hands on your ribcage and breathe in wide and deep, filling your lungs with air. Imagine your lungs are a pair of bellows. Feel your ribcage expanding as your lungs fill with air and your diaphragm lowers, then breathe the air out thorough your mouth. The wider and deeper you breathe in, the more fresh air you take in to oxygenate your blood. As you breathe out, try to exhale all the air you have taken in and you will find that, as your lungs empty, your diaphragm will start to rise and this, in turn, will help you connect your deep abdominal muscles from your navel through to your spine.

Where a Pilates movement demands most effort, use your out-breath to maximum effect.

Not only will thoracic breathing allow you to move more effectively in Pilates, but it will also help focus your mind on the movement as you take the time to concentrate on your own body.

Flowing Movement

After spending hours perfecting your trot-canter transitions at home to ensure you and horse are a picture of flowing movement when you enter the dressage arena at A, so you need to flow and demonstrate easy progressions and harmony when you are practising Pilates.

As with learning anything new, be patient; flow will develop the more you practise, until it becomes second nature. It takes some time to develop, but the stronger your centre becomes, the easier it will be to move your arms and legs out from a stable core in a flowing, easy-looking movement. Just think back to how it was when you first learnt shoulder-in or tried jumping down a grid. It was probably a bit mechanical and jerky as you tried to remember all your aids in the right place – when to sit, when to fold forward, or when to move your horse forward with your seat.

As you become more practised, you will become more confident as you move your body through all planes of movement such as flexion, extension, lateral flexion and rotation.

Alignment, Co-ordination and Precision

Alignment, co-ordination and precision of the body when in motion are the building blocks of Pilates and should be reflected upon regularly during a session, so as to enjoy the full effect of the movement and achieve balance in a co-ordinated way. You need to ensure that your body is in alignment before you even think about moving. As a beginner, ask yourself every time you finish a movement: 'Am I level, straight; are my pelvis and spine in neutral; are my legs like tramlines to enable my body to move efficiently for maximum effect?' This checklist will soon become second

nature. Precision and awareness of your body are essential to perfecting each and every Pilates movement. If thinking in terms of equitation, think of these principles as 'feel'.

Relaxation and Concentration

Relaxation and concentration may appear to be almost opposites, but they both apply equally to Pilates. These two traits probably come easier to a rider as, to be successful in the saddle, you must be relaxed in your body to convey authority and leadership to your horse, but equally you need to concentrate your mind, especially if you are riding around a showjumping course or remembering complex movements in a dressage test. Tension is not an option!

When scheduling-in a Pilates session, make sure it is at a time of day when you can concentrate fully on what you are doing and put everything else out of your mind, rather than manically squashing it into the half-hour break between the vet and the farrier! Allow yourself this time – it is your time to concentrate on strengthening your own body. Think of it as making a bank deposit in a high-interest account. The deposit is your time spent doing the exercises; your reward is the interest – your fitter, stronger body you accumulate and can 'cash in' on a rainy day. The rainy day being when you are full steam ahead on the showjumping or eventing circuit and need extra strength and conditioning to get yourself through. You worry enough about your horse's needs – it is now time to concentrate on your own. By putting aside a regular slot – whether it is fifteen minutes a day before breakfast or half an hour after evening stables four times a week – you will see your own body strengthening markedly and improving in tone and your mind benefiting from the relaxation Pilates offers.

Stamina

Just as you wouldn't go to an event two weeks after bringing your horse in from the field following his winter break, don't expect to be doing advanced Pilates a few weeks after you start! When you bring your horse in, you start with gentle walking and roadwork to build up muscle and stamina – the same goes for you.

It is important to build up your muscles slowly, as you are working on the deep postural muscles rather than the large muscles responsible for big movements such as walking. This way, you will build muscle memory. In Pilates the emphasis is on *quality* of movement – think back to the principles of alignment, co-ordination and precision – rather than *quantity*. Pilates is not about exercising until you drop or pushing yourself until you are physically and mentally exhausted – leave that to the gym bunnies!

You don't need to sweat and feel fatigued to convince yourself you have completed a worthwhile Pilates session. If you ride for a living then, as an athlete, you may feel you want to add in a different cardiovascular exercise such as swimming or running to complement your Pilates workouts if you feel riding several horses a day is not enough. However, think in the same terms as when you are teaching a horse a new movement, such as half-pass – you don't ask for the movement repeatedly for the whole forty

minutes you are riding – you weave it into a horse's programme along with other learnt movements and revisit it over a period of time until you have perfected it together.

Mind-body

As well as strengthening your body, Pilates does a power of good for your mental well-being, too. Your mind and body are connected – if you feel good physically, then your demeanour improves. If you have in your mind's eye a poor body image of yourself, it often follows that you will harbour negative thoughts. Certain exercises – especially those that target muscle groups where we tend to hold tension, such as the shoulders, ribs and spine – can instantly give you a mental lift. So next time you are feeling low, try Arm Openings, Tree Hugging, Spine Curl, Roll Down, Lumbar Stretch, Shoulder Drops, Cobra, Dart and Rest Position.

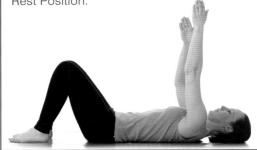

Rider Attributes
Proprioception
Balance
Control
Focus
Rhythm

Your Pilates Aids

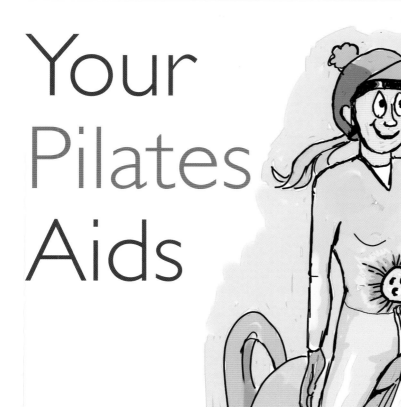

Zip-up

Just as you would use a sequence of aids when asking your horse to half-halt to ensure the best engagement, lift and balance him to set him up for the next movement, so in Pilates you need to implement the following two aids to stabilise your core before you move.

The first aid is the lifting up of the pelvic floor – and yes, guys can do this, too! If you have been to a Pilates session or watched a Pilates DVD, you would have heard the instructor asking you to 'zip-up' your pelvic floor muscles, which to the uninitiated sounds like torture! If you are not sure how to engage or locate your pelvic floor, let alone its muscles, think of what you would do to stop urinating in mid-flow. It is this feeling of drawing up inside that engages the pelvic floor muscles which are so essential for core stability. If you are still in the dark, then imagine how you would stop yourself from passing wind in a packed secretary's tent, and it is this reaction you need to engage! Try drawing up this imaginary zip from the back passage through to the front! Very glamorous, but well-worth the effort!

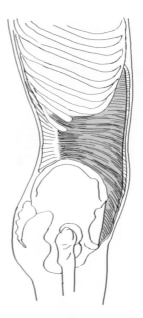

Transversus abdominis muscle

Navel to Spine

Some teachers use the instruction, 'sinking your navel through to your spine'; others would say 'hollow your tummy' or 'engage your abdominals', 'powerhouse' or 'core'. All basically mean to draw in your tummy muscles, as if you were pulling them through to your back. Picture your trunk and think of it as a mattress. The mattress button that fixes the front through to the back is your transversus abdominis muscle, which attaches to your lower ribs and down to your pelvis at the front of your body, passes through your middle and attaches to your spine, back of your ribs and pelvis in your lower back. This muscle creates a corset of strength around your middle and is the muscle we are going to recruit to help build your core stability.

Collective of Both Aids

In this book, the collective of both the above aids will be the instruction to 'stabilise', which will mean to draw up your pelvic floor and then engage your deep abdominals.

Core Stability

You know yourself that if you are lungeing a fresh horse who suddenly takes fright, unless you can quickly and effectively ground yourself you will be caught off balance which, at best, can lead to a pulled muscle, or at worst you can be dragged across the arena. This is because, while it is easy to depend on the big moving muscles for brute strength, the secret of strength is actually in the recruitment of the smaller, deep, stabilising muscles of the torso to act quickly and protect the body.

When mounted, having control through your body will help you to influence your horse in a subtle way. With control of your core you can go up and down the 'gears', change gait, shorten and lengthen strides, encourage your mount forward and check, all with slight movements – or 'engaging' of – your deep core muscles.

There are three main areas of the body where a rider needs to be flexible but strong, stable yet mobile – these are the pelvis, lower back (lumbar spine) and upper body, including the thoracic spine and shoulders. These are the three core areas this book will concentrate on with regard to building stability through Pilates exercises.

Pelvic Stability

In a rider, the tell-tale sign of pelvic instability is the inability to keep the torso stable when the horse is moving, so the rider's legs and arms move uncontrollably. As a rider you need to be able to keep you pelvis stable and level whilst the legs either stay still on the horse's sides, or you move them independently of one another in a controlled manner when giving your aids. To do this successfully, you need to engage the pelvic floor muscles – which accounts for the lifting or the 'zip' command, and also to engage the transversus abdominis muscle, which, as mentioned earlier, is essentially the main muscle which, along with several other smaller muscles, connects your front to your back. But the main players in pelvic stability for a rider are the gluteus medius, a pair of deep muscles which are located one each side at your hips and which attach to the top of the femur at their base and around the lip of the hip bone.

A common rider problem is a weakness of the gluteus medius muscles. If they are weak on both sides, then a rider can suffer from tight hamstrings as this large muscle will take

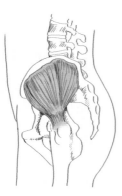

on a stabilising, rather than a mobilising role. If the gluteus medius is weak on one side, then another muscle on the opposite side, the quadratus lumborum, kicks in, working overtime to try to help stabilise the pelvis. The result is that the rider hitches up their hip on one side and this means a shortening of one leg and dropping down of the hip – leading to a crooked

Gluteus medius muscle

rider with an uneven distribution of weight on the horse's back, plus the added insecurity of balance being compromised.

Lumbar Spine Stability

Think of your spine as a stack of building bricks, placed one of top of another from your pelvis to your head.

To keep the lumbar spine stable whilst you move, once you are in neutral with all your natural curves in your lower back (not pressed or flattened into the mat) you need to lift up your pelvic floor muscles and engage your muscles from your navel through to your spine. The muscles you will engage are the transversus abdominis, pelvic floor and the multifidus, the small muscles like cocktail sausages that run the length of your spine and help keep you upright. Other abdominal muscles which help to stabilise the spine during various planes of movement are the rectus abdominis, a muscle divided into several 'bellies' commonly known as the 'six pack', which help you flex and also tilt the

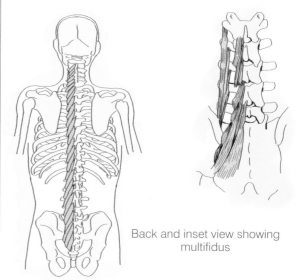

Back and inset view showing multifidus

pelvis, and the internal and external oblique muscles, which help with rotation and lateral or side flexion of the body.

A supple lumbar spine will enable you to drive from your seat (as appropriate), therefore encouraging your horse to be supple through his spine and in turn, swing beneath you. If a horse is tense through his back, the rider will bounce in the saddle. The horse and rider should be as one. If you, as the rider, brace your back, the horse will do the same and tighten his – the horse is like a mirror and will reflect what he feels from his rider. Relaxed rider, relaxed horse.(Regarding the terms 'brace' and 'bracing', I am mindful that some schools of equitation have, in the past, used these terms not to describe undue stiffness but in the context of legitimate and effective 'holding' and 'pushing' aids. I should therefore make it clear that, within this text, the terms 'brace' and 'bracing' are used to convey an undue level of stiffness and tension that will always be counterproductive when riding.)

Realxed rider, relaxed horse.

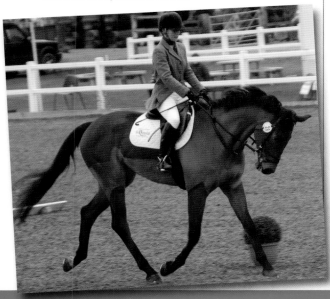

Neutral Pelvis and Neutral Spine

When working through Pilates exercises, it is essential to ensure that you are working from a neutral pelvis and neutral spine position. A neutral pelvis is one where you are neither tipped forward nor back, or more to one side than the other – rather your body rests 'naturally' in the middle. One of the easiest ways to find neutral is from Relaxation Position (see page 52). Neutral spine is where you allow for all the normal, natural curves of your spine in all positions and, for example, you neither flatten them into the mat when working from relaxation position, nor arch your back unnaturally the other way to perform any movements.

Shoulder (Scapular) Stability

As a rider, the stability of your upper body is key to your balance and harmony in the saddle. One of the most valuable Pilates sequences learnt by riders is the ability to relax the shoulder-blades down the back and thus stabilise the shoulder girdle, something which, following practice of various Pilates exercises, soon becomes second nature, not only when on a horse but during everyday activity. Bingo! Dressage marks improve radically as the upper body is given lift and elegance! Jumpers benefit from increased stability and balance in the saddle with a fantastic ability to sit up with more effect, either between fences on a course or as a safety net when caught unawares across country.

As a consequence of the shoulder-blades relaxing down the back, the neck lengthens, gently elongating the spine and making you feel taller.

Stabiliser and Mobiliser Muscles

This is not intended to be an anatomy book so the explanation of muscle strength and weakness will be brief. To simplify muscle activity, think of all muscles as operating either to stabilise or mobilise. Technically, all muscles have some 'stability role'. A mobiliser muscle, such as a hamstring, makes big, whole limb movements. These big muscles work in phases as they can tire very easily. They are usually located near the surface of the body and tend to be long muscles, whereas a stabiliser or postural muscle is located deeper in the body, facilitates endurance by working for long periods at a time and holds tone.

If you are carrying an injury or have poor posture, the stabilising muscles elongate and become weak. Muscles that have a predominantly stabilising role will then either become long and weak or short, tight and weak. If you don't use them at all, they will waste. As you become less mobile as you 'protect' your injury by not using the underlying muscles – and therefore do not rely on the deep postural muscles for stability – you will find that the mobilising muscles take on the role of the stabilisers.

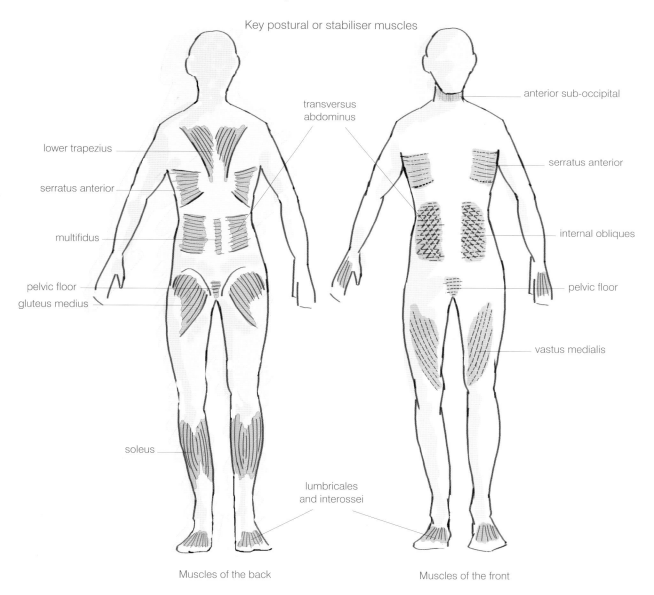

Key postural or stabiliser muscles

transversus abdominus

lower trapezius

serratus anterior

multifidus

pelvic floor

gluteus medius

soleus

lumbricales and interossei

anterior sub-occipital

serratus anterior

internal obliques

pelvic floor

vastus medialis

Muscles of the back

Muscles of the front

Muscle Imbalances and Weaknesses

It is a well-known fact that in the arena, many riders 'cheat' to make themselves look good in front of the judges. I don't mean that they bribed the judges – far from it!! No, they cheat by using their body incorrectly to cover up issues they may have, whether it is a painful nagging injury, a stiffness or a muscle weakness. Instead of using the stabilising muscles to support their core and be strong from the inside out, they use their big, mobilising muscles.

If a rider is carrying an injury, then a mobilising muscle will take over the role of a weakened stabilising muscle. If, for example, a rider is on the showjumping circuit for eight weeks at a time, with little time for themselves, this will cause muscle fatigue and further weakness, plunging the rider into a downward spiral and minimising their effectiveness in the saddle, which leads to dissatisfaction and in some cases, further injury.

Many riders have imbalances and don't realise it. For example, does your horse feel better balanced on the right rein than the left? Do you feel more comfortable jumping on the left rein rather than the right? Did you think your horse was at fault? In fact, this could be your influence over him, which may have built up over time, especially if you are a one-horse rider (See Crookedness, page 38). Weak muscles can be anywhere from your neck down to your feet, and everywhere in between! The important thing is to work on your weaknesses first before strengthening muscles. Pick exercises that allow you to work in all planes of movement so that you can rebalance your body evenly and gain strength around your core – which will, in turn, increase your independent limb control and fight off fatigue. Generally there are three types of rider imbalances as detailed below.

Tight One Side with Opposite Side Weak

This is the most common. Many riders collapse through their waist and hip, lengthen one leg and drop their shoulder. They will look uneven in the saddle, and maybe even give the appearance that they have one stirrup leather longer than the other. Here, the transversus abdominis, gluteus muscles, latissimus dorsi and abdominals are under-active.

● Key Exercises
Curl-ups
Leg Circles and the series of leg exercises
Thread the Needle
Arm Openings

Weak on Both Sides

The tell-tale sign of this is excessive movement on both sides of the body. The rider may suffer lower back (lumbar) and upper back (thoracic) pain, owing to their exaggerated movements. This is often a complaint of a tall rider with long limbs.

● Key Exercises
Spine Curl
Diamond Press
Cobra
Compass
Table Top

Tight and Weak on Same Side

Here, a mobilising muscle may have taken on the role of a stabilising one, which is very often because of an injury. It is important to focus on exercises that target lateral stability and the gluteus medius and piriformis muscle.

● Key Exercises
Roll Downs

Hip Rolls
Oblique Curl-ups
Oyster
Side Reach

Lumbar Spine Stiffness

How often do you get off your horse, arching your lower back to get some relief from the stiffness? Have you ever sat at home at night following a day of competition, wishing you hadn't done quite as much? Back pain is really common among riders and contributes to fatigue and repetitive injury if left unchecked.

Abdominal muscle tone contributes to the stability of the lumbar spine. If this is weak, injuries occur. The transversus abdominis muscle acts like a 'corset' – it connects to other spinal structures to form a corset-like structure. Strengthening this important muscle, in partnership with the multifidus along your spine and your 'six pack' muscle (rectus abdominis) and the pelvic floor muscles, will help to keep the lower back protected.

Having a supple lumbar spine means that you will be able to influence your horse better with your seat. Your horse will then mirror this and begin to swing through his back. If you are tense or brace through your back, maybe trying to 'protect' an injury, your horse will stiffen and maybe shorten his stride. A rider with a stiff lower back will bounce in the saddle.

● Key Exercises
Spine Curl with Arms
The Cat
Rest Position

Tight Hip Flexors

One of the most frequent problems for a rider is tight hip flexors, mainly arising from the riding position. The legs are constantly bent at the knee with the foot flexed in the stirrup. The pelvis and upper thigh are 'held' in the saddle, with the hips and knees bent. The psoas group of muscles allows the knee and thigh to bend up towards the waist and it is important to stretch these muscles out. They attach the thigh bone to the lower back and if they are tight, you may suffer a hollow lower back, or lordosis.

Tight hip flexors can be agony! To release these muscles, incorporate the following exercises into your Pilates workout.

● Key Exercises
Hip Flexor Stretch
Single Leg Stretch

Tight Hamstrings

Another frequent rider complaint is tight hamstrings. These are the group of three long muscles located along the back of the thigh, attached to the back of the knee, which flex and bend the knee. Again, sitting behind a desk or constantly sitting in the riding position doesn't help. Short, tight hamstrings can be painful, so to keep comfortable it is important to stretch them little and often. Try adding the following exercises into your Pilates workout.

● Key Exercises
Hamstring Stretch
Battement
The series of leg exercises

Common Rider Complaints

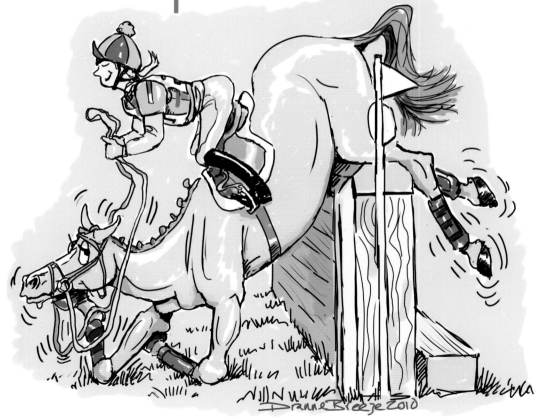

The following are general issues that will have an adverse effect on riding effectively.

Crookedness

Beware – crookedness could be triggered by the horse who may have developed more muscle on one side than the other; by the rider from an old or recent injury, or very often it can be caused by the saddle with less flocking in one side than the other, or a twist in the tree following damage from a drop, or fall of horse and rider.

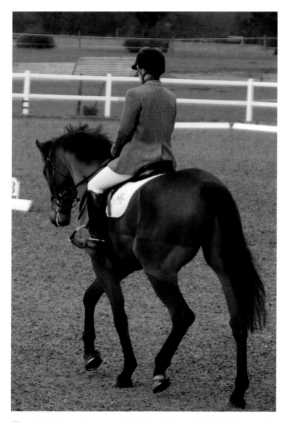

The rider's spine needs to be in a straight line and directly above the horse's spine.

Remember – your horse is a mirror. If your weight is unevenly distributed, or if you are stronger on one side than the other, the horse will reflect this as he tries to counterbalance the load – you. Riders particularly cannot afford muscle imbalances as these show up very clearly in the dressage arena. As soon as these creep in, you will find that your horse appears to go better on one rein than the other.

● Key Exercises

To alleviate crookedness, try adding the following Front-lying exercises into your Pilates workout:

Diamond Press
Dart
Cobra
Oyster

Tips!

When in the saddle, try gently rolling your tailbone under you, which will help engage your pelvic floor muscles which, in turn, will help you become more effective with your seat.

Try breathing wide and deep into the sides of your ribcage when walking on a free rein. Horses can often jog when asked to execute this movement, purely because of rider tension. By relaxing into the walk, and feeling your shoulder-blades slide down your back, you should feel any tension melt away and your horse should respond by stretching down further.

Bracing and Tension

Engaging your core muscles does not mean bracing to the extent of producing undue tension and stiffness. That is why Pilates movements are executed as you breathe out. Breathing methods are central to the Pilates system as, if tense, a rider's posture will change, become protective, closed and hunched, whilst breathing becomes rapid and shallow. Taking deep, wide breaths into the ribcage slows your breathing and allows your body to move freely and without tension; filling the lungs with oxygen relaxes you and in turn gives you more vigour and energy.

● Key Exercises

To alleviate tension, try adding the following exercises into your Pilates workout:

Shoulder Drops
Thread the Needle
Spine Curls
Dart
Rest Position

Excessive Arm and Leg Movement

By making your own centre stronger, as you build up your corset of strength by engaging your transversus abdominis, rectus abdominis and pelvic floor muscles, you will be able control and move your arms and legs independently.

Remember the words 'independent seat' shouted at you since you were a child trotting around the arena? Well, it is nigh on impossible to do this without first engaging, or centring your powerhouse so that you can free up the rest of your body to move without tension.

You will often see riders – and not just beginners – with poor postural stability trying to stay central in the saddle, over-compensating by constantly shifting their arms and legs.

● Key Exercises

To improve core stability, try adding the following exercises into your Pilates workout:

Spine Curls
Curl-ups
Knee Folds
Single Leg Stretch

Neck or Upper Body Stiffness

A lot of tension can be carried in the shoulders and neck. Rapid or shallow breathing can lead to neck stiffness or muscle imbalance in the upper back, which can easily lead to tiredness and pain. Instead of reaching for the anti-inflammatories, try doing a few simple Pilates exercises.

● Key Exercises

Shoulder Drops and Tree Hugging may replace the need for anti-inflammatories. Also, try adding the following exercises into your Pilates workout:

Yes and No Neck Tucks and Rolls
Hip Rolls
Dart
Diamond Press
Cobra

Directions of Movement

Just as you school your horse on both reins, allow him time to be long and low, gently bend his head and neck and ask him to respond to your leg aids to bend or be straight and thus achieve suppleness, so you need to allow yourself to move in all directions and not become fixed in just one plane of movement. For example, you wouldn't jump on your horse and ask for instant collection – if you did, you would end up with a very stiff horse!

Pilates recognises the need for movement in all directions so exercises can be generally split into rotation, lateral flexion, flexion and extension, with some combination movements. If you have a particular problem area you would like to target, have a look at the list on page 42.

Rotation

Hip Rolls
Arm Openings
Waist Twist

Lateral Flexion

Side Reach

Flexion

Roll Down
Curl-ups
Single Leg Stretch

The Hundred
Spine Curl with Arms
Roll Backs
Cat
Studio Stretch

Extension

Dart
Diamond Press
Cobra
Single Leg Kick

Combination Movements

Thread the Needle
Rolling Like a Ball
Oblique Curl-ups

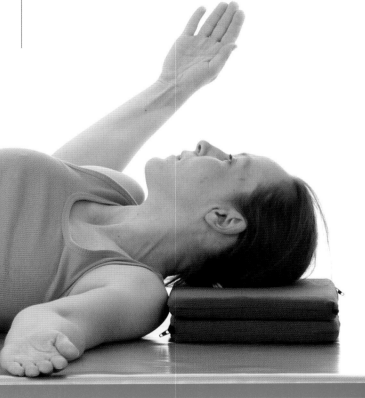

Targeted Exercises

The following is a summary of exercises that target development of particular areas of the body. They are all explained fully in the pages that follow.

Upper Body

Yes and No Neck Rolls and Chin Tucks
Tree Hugging
Shoulder Drops
Diamond Press
Dart
Ribcage Closure
Backstroke Swimming

Lower Body/Pelvic Stability

(To help develop an independent seat)
Backstroke Swimming
Knee Drops
Knee Folds
Knee Stirs
Leg Circles
Table Top

Standing on One Leg
Oyster
Compass

Leg/Bottom Exercises

Oyster
Side-lying Leg Lifts
Side-lying Leg Circles
Side-lying Inner Thigh Lift
Side-lying Legs Flex Forward

Rider Stretches

Hamstring Stretch
Hip Flexor Stretch
Studio Stretch
Gluteus and Piriformis Stretch

Your Posture

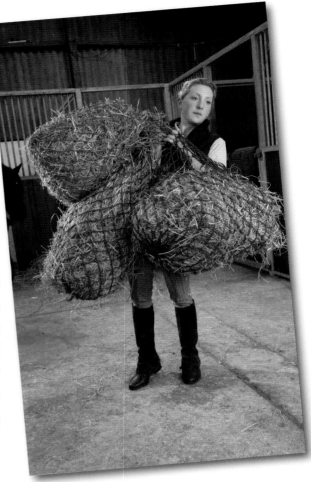

The wrong way to carry haynets

Your posture is so important both on and off the horse. When mounted and competing, it can mean the difference between a 5 and an 8 in the dressage, or a near miss or fall when jumping, as it is intrinsically linked to stability and balance in the saddle.

Every one of us has a slightly different posture and can also have several different postural faults. As children, we are born with a near-perfect posture. Toddlers sit so upright and open through the chest when playing on the floor because they are recruiting their deep postural muscles to stay upright. This is before all the hang-ups of modern life take their toll, such as heavy school bags, sitting hunched over a desk, or an ill-sized chair. If not corrected, this situation can spiral downwards as we add in sitting crouched over a computer desk all day with our arms constantly in front of us, elongating the muscles which should be shorter in order to give support in our upper back and shoulders. Then, after a day's work, we rush to the yard in the car – another hunched position – where we throw ourselves headlong into yard work such as carrying heavy soaked haynets, wheel overfilled wheelbarrows, waddle unevenly loaded with

A better way to move haynets

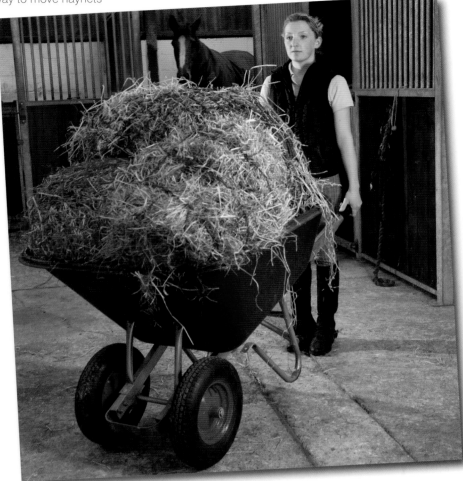

buckets and heavy bales of hay or shavings, throw up heavy lorry ramps and lead out feisty youngsters to the field – is it any wonder that a rider's posture can leave a lot to be desired, with pain and aching backs the 'norm'? Repeated bad movements and overusing the same muscles leads to stiffness because of tight muscles.

But it is not too late to do something about it. The good news is that the more you tell your body to move in a certain way by practicing Pilates, the more it 'remembers' that movement pattern. You will also become more body-aware and correct yourself. This amended movement then becomes your natural, normal movement and your body as a whole becomes more flowing and free.

Generally, we fall into four broad categories of postural faults, but we can also have a mixture of all four, much of it depending on our lifestyle.

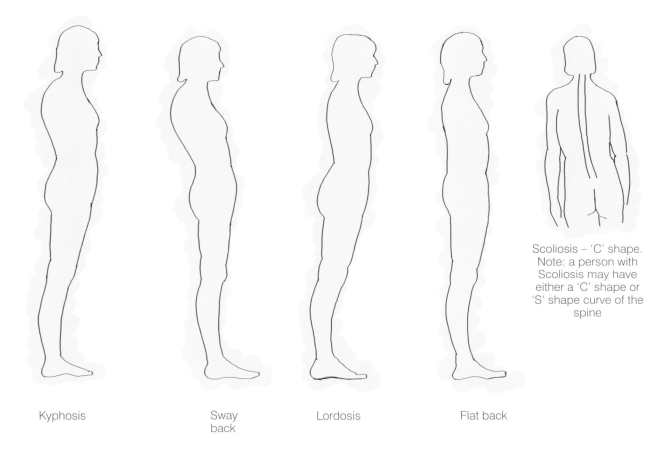

Scoliosis – 'C' shape. Note: a person with Scoliosis may have either a 'C' shape or 'S' shape curve of the spine

Kyphosis

Sway back

Lordosis

Flat back

Kyphosis

A person with a kyphosis is identified by an exaggerated doming of the upper back, around the thoracic area of the spine, giving a round-shouldered look. This can be caused by permanently hunched shoulders – perhaps related to contact through the reins where the arms are permanently forward without the benefit of the shoulder-blades being drawn down the back. Also, the pectoral muscles (located at the front of the body, attached to the clavicles, sternum, ribs and upper arms) may feel tight.

● Three Key Exercises
Roll Downs
Shoulder Drops
Arm Openings

Lordosis

Quite common among riders, a lordotic posture is one where the lower back is hollow, or arched. Sitting on a horse for long periods can mean that the hip flexors become tight and the lower abdominal muscles and bottom, or gluteals, become weak. A by-product of weak gluteals is that the hamstrings, a group of muscles responsible for big movements, take over the stabilising role of the gluteus medius

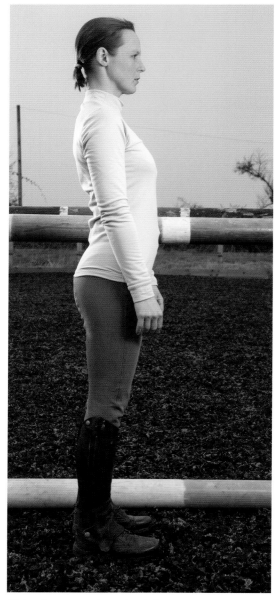

Rider demonstrating a lordotic posture

and become tight and restrained. This then allows the pelvis to tip forward, increasing the hollow in the lower back.

- Three Key Exercises
  Hip Rolls
  Curl-ups
  The Hundred

Sway Back

This can be another common rider postural fault, particularly among young teenage riders! Here the pelvis is tipped forward, so the rider looks to be 'hanging' or sitting on their hips. Their abdomen is pushed out in front of them, with an increased curve or hollow in the lower spine, plus a doming of the upper back.

- Three Key Exercises
  Hamstring Stretch
  Side Reach
  Single Leg Stretch

Flat Back

Looking at a flat back sideways on, there will be little or indeed no curve in the lower back. The pelvis will also be tilted backwards, rather than in neutral. The bottom will have little or no tone or lift and the head will be poking forwards. The rider may also suffer from tight hamstrings.

- Three Key Exercises
  Single Leg Stretch
  Oblique Curl-ups
  The Cat

Added Benefits of Pilates

Greater joint mobility
Fewer headaches (where they are posture-based)
Boosted immune system
Lowered stress levels
More efficient lymphatic system
Better respiratory system

As well as helping to develop improved feel, pilates builds greater confidence in the saddle

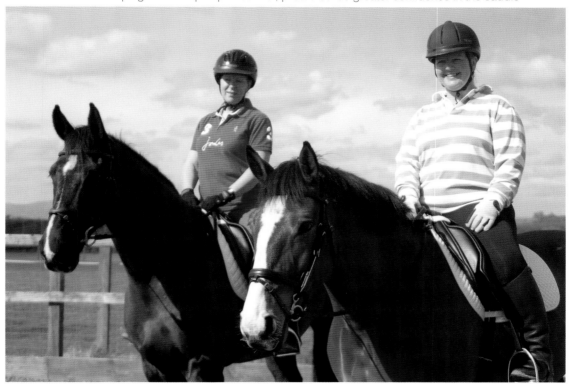

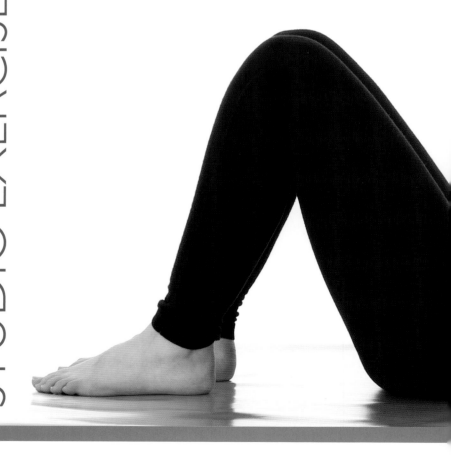

PART TWO
STUDIO EXERCISES

Key Pilates Starting Positions

There are several key positions that form the starting points for Pilates exercises. Before going on to describe the exercises in detail, below is a brief explanation of the 'whys and hows' of these individual positions.

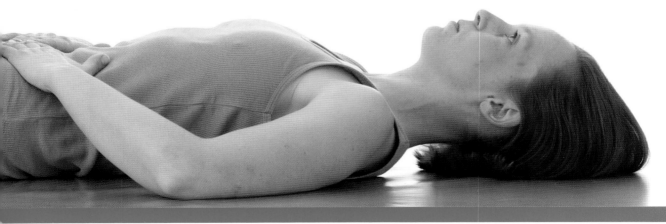

Standing Correctly

Why?

When standing we are challenging gravity, which makes it an exercise in its own right. Standing correctly will not only use the deep postural muscles, but is a great exercise to create muscle memory, so once you've practised it by running through the method below, you will find that you start to do this more naturally in everyday life without even thinking about it! Think how much taller you will sit on your horse after this simple exercise. Enjoy!

How?

Stand with your feet placed squarely on the floor – almost feel as if you are pushing the ground away from you – this will help you stand tall. Imagine someone has hold of your hair on the top of your head and is pulling it up towards the ceiling. Think of lengthening the distance from your neck to your shoulders, feel your collarbones widening and your shoulder-blades sliding down your back. Banish those round shoulders and think tall! Lengthen through your waist, feeling the distance increasing from the bottom of your ribs to your hips. Gently draw up the pelvic floor and feel the engagement through the abdominals – breathe! Soften at the knees without bracing, lift your upper body and feel the weight of your body evenly distributed through your feet, from your big toes right through to your little toes and your heels. Memorise this feeling of connection, remembering how you are standing and how your muscles are recruited.

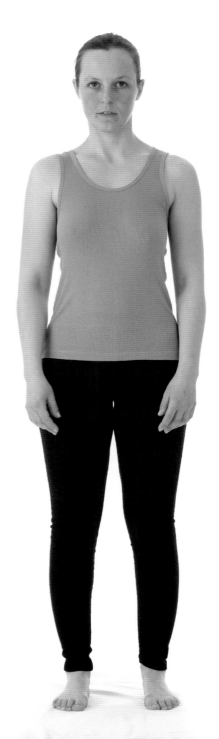

Pilates Stance

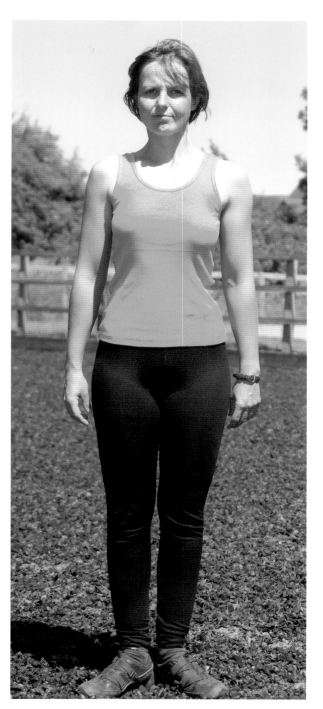

Why?

Pilates stance is a step on from standing correctly. As well as challenging gravity, getting all the little, deep muscles to work, it taps into the inner thigh and deep gluteal muscles which will help later as you try out some of the more advanced exercises.

How?

Follow the instructions on page 50 for standing correctly, but with your heels together and feet rotated slightly outwards – remember your ballet lessons as a child and how wonderfully you stood in first position! The rotation is of the whole legs from the hips – not just a rotation of the knees or ankles. Also feel the connection between the inner thighs by gently drawing them together. Feel strong and connected throughout your body as one unit. Again, remember how this feels with your deep postural muscles active.

Relaxation Position

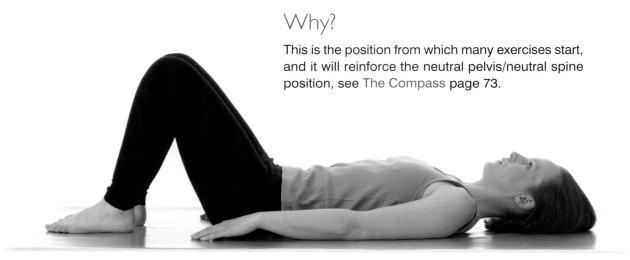

Why?

This is the position from which many exercises start, and it will reinforce the neutral pelvis/neutral spine position, see The Compass page 73.

How?

Lie on your back with your feet hip-width apart and parallel, feet flat, making contact with the floor, knees raised, hips feeling heavy as if they are dropping into your hip sockets and through the mat below. Feel the weight of your head, upper body and pelvis melting into the mat. Relax! Find a position where your pelvis and spine are in neutral position; pelvis not tipped forwards or back, but in the middle, with hip bones parallel to the ceiling and your spine with all its natural curves, not flattened into the mat. Breathe wide and deep into your ribcage, as if your lungs are a pair of bellows, filling with air. Breathe in through your nose and out through your mouth.

Gently stabilise on your out-breath before moving.

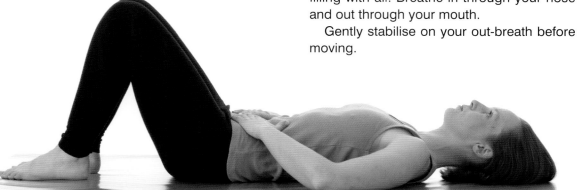

Front-lying or Prone

Why?

Lying on your tummy, or in prone position, you can more easily work your back extensor muscles and your shoulder girdle, so that you can isolate and improve your upper body stability.

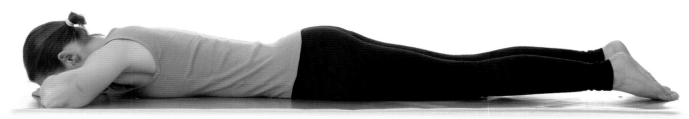

How?

When lying on your front, it is easy to collapse the body into the mat and just lie there as though you were sunning yourself in the Caribbean! It is important to think of the mat as an exercise tool and therefore you need to 'oppose' it. This means that you need to keep your body active, for example by drawing up your pelvic floor and engaging your tummy muscles, by lengthening your waist and challenging the mat with your ribcage and feeling tall and lengthened in your body from the top of your head to the tips of your toes. Feel that your hips are open and that your spine is allowed its natural curves, neither flattened nor arched on the mat. Give yourself a few seconds to release through the shoulders and feel that your collarbones are gently widening.

Four-point Kneeling

Why?

It is important to work with a neutral pelvis and spine in all Pilates positions, to help you become stronger through your core and challenge your body in positions that defy gravity! As a rider, this is also a challenge for your upper body and shoulders, and helps create scapular stability (see page 31). Upper body stability helps create mobility elsewhere, which is essential for achieving grace and precision when riding.

How?

With your knees and hands on the floor, position yourself so that your hands are directly under your shoulders and your arms are straight but not rigid. Connect your shoulders lightly, in such a way that your shoulder-blades are drawn down your back, but without bracing. Have your knees directly below your hips. Check behind to ensure that your feet, lower legs and thighs are aligned, like tramlines. Allow your neck to have its natural curves, feeling long and looking down towards the mat. Feel the strength from your centre and stabilise.

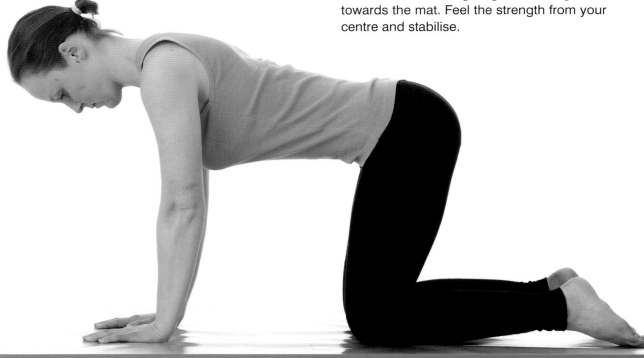

Side-lying

Why?

Many exercises (for example Oyster, Leg Series) that target the gluteus medius, a muscle that is central to achieving pelvic stability, are performed in side-lying. Also, further challenges are placed on the body in side-lying with the addition of rotation exercises, such as Arm Openings.

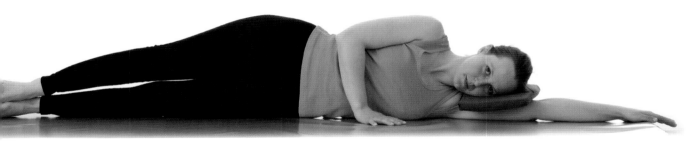

How?

Each exercise will instruct whether to lie with arms out in front of you or above you, with your head resting on your lower arm, but essentially the principles are the same. Lie on your side with your waist long on both sides; do this by stretching out the gap between your bottom rib and your hips, by reaching out further with your leg. Ensure that your hips are stacked one on top of the other and that your pelvis is square and in neutral, not tipping forward or falling backwards. Stretch out your legs so that they are lengthening from your hip sockets through to your heels – this will greatly assist you when you need to lengthen your legs when mounted.

Sitting

Why?

One of the most essential positions to perfect as you are sitting for most of the time, unless you are jumping or riding with a two-point seat across country, or racing.

How?

Exercises such as The Saw and Studio Stretches are performed sitting, but with legs in varying positions (see individual exercises for exact leg positioning).

As in standing, achieving length in your spine is the most important thing, so sit tall on your seat bones and imagine your lower back is like a bungee and gently stretch it upwards. Feel yourself sit taller as you breathe in and lift yourself up further as if someone is pulling your hair up towards the ceiling; elongate your neck and feel the gap widening between your ears and shoulders. Stabilise through your centre, and lengthen up along your waist. Lift the ribcage, but do not flare or brace it. Ensure that your ribcage is above your pelvis, not slumped forwards or tilted backwards. You can help yourself do this by allowing your shoulder-blades to rest down your back, which will, in turn, widen your collarbones at the front of your body.

A Note on the 'C' Curve

Learning to work in a 'C' curve position in Pilates will help you when you are in the saddle, as you will be able to mobilise your pelvis easily, so that it can, for example, better act as a shock-absorber when jumping. You will also be able to move with the horse rather than act as a block to his movement through your seat. The 'C' curve is a natural position for the lower spine and you can see how to create that position by looking at, for example, the Roll Back (page 162).

Studio Exercise Programme

I n the following pages you will find a detailed explanation of each exercise from the different starting positions of Standing, Relaxation, Front-lying, Four-point Kneeling, Side-lying and Sitting. For the best mind-body workout, pick one or two from each starting positing and vary them daily, as even though each starts from the same position, they may encompass different movements, for example in Standing, the Roll Down concentrates on bending the spine forwards (flexion), whereas Waist Twist encompasses twisting (rotation).

If you feel you have a bit of a problem area that you would like to work on, increase the number of exercises that target that specific area, for example, if you feel you tip forward in the saddle, add in Ribcage Closure and Hip Flexor Stretch. But bear in mind that, to achieve the best results in Pilates, your workout should include a variety of exercises that challenge the body in all areas, so that you rebalance the whole of the body.

Every exercise is colour-flagged to indicate its challenge level, and it's important to include a variety of levels in each workout. On the exercise scale, the easier movements are flagged orange, then pink, with more intermediate exercises yellow, moving through to green and then red, which require more core stability. Include more orange, pink and yellow exercises in the first few weeks, moving up to adding in one or two green then a couple of red, if you feel comfortable with your level of stability. The number of repetitions is written in the flag.

Each exercise also has a Why? box where you will find an explanation of how it helps the body, plus the equestrian advantage it gives.

You can further increase the challenge and change the dynamics of your workout as your stability grows by adding in some of the optional extras, which are progressions of the exercises.

Time to Exercise!

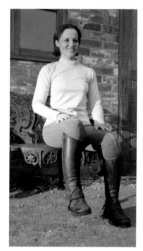

With Pilates, little or no equipment is necessary and you can do your workout inside or out. Little and often is best. If you only have time to do one or two exercises a day, don't worry, as it will be hugely beneficial in the long run. If you don't have a Pilates mat, use a rug or towel instead. A folded-up towel makes an excellent head cushion. If you don't have a flexi-band, a scarf will do. Don't let a lack of equipment today delay the start of your programme until tomorrow!

Exercise Scale

Orange – beginner

Pink – improver

Yellow – more challenging

Green – intermediate

Red – advanced

As with any form of exercise, please do not attempt the programme if you are injured in any way. If you have suffered a recent fall or are carrying an injury, ensure you are cleared to exercise by your doctor.

Exercises from Standing

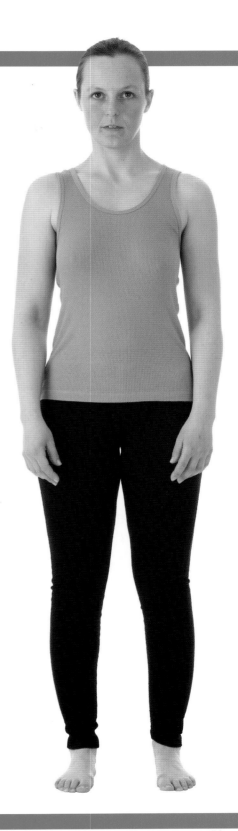

Dumb Waiter 6x

Why?

To open the upper body and collarbone area
and strengthen the shoulder stabilisers and
rotator muscles.

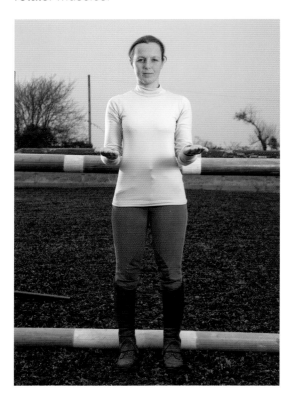 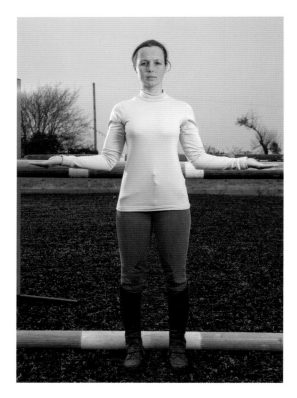

How?

From Standing (see page 50), open your
arms out in front of you with palms open,
elbows under shoulders, as if carrying a just-
cleaned bridle. Your elbows are by your sides,
but not forced or bracing. Stabilise, and as

you breathe in and lengthen through your
spine, open your arms out to the side, feeling
the movement start and rotate from your
shoulders, not your elbows. As you breathe
out, return to the starting position.

Roll Down 8x

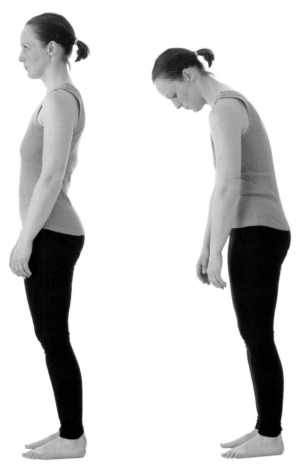

Why?

To release tension in the upper body and create flexibility, whilst strengthening the back, bottom and legs.

Equestrian Advantage

Mobilises the spine and hips and achieves segmental control of the spine

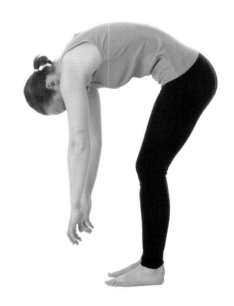

How?

From Standing in a lengthened position, arms at your sides, on your out-breath stabilise and nod your head, soften through your breastbone and start to roll the body forwards, feeling the segmental movement through each vertebra. Bend or soften at the knee to avoid straining the muscles at the back of your legs (hamstrings). Allow the arms to hang. Take a wide, deep breath into the sides of your ribcage, then, initiating the movement with your pelvis, on your out-breath, start to re-stack the body, bone by bone, until you are back at the starting position.

Tennis Ball Rising 8x ▷

Why?

Strengthens the bottom, thigh and calf muscles and mobilises ankles and feet.

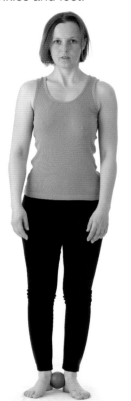
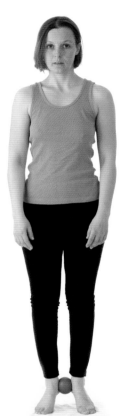
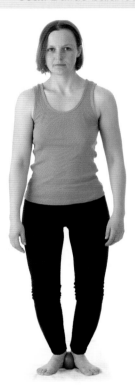

How?

Place a tennis ball between your ankles, just below the inside ankle bones. From Standing, inhale and lengthen then, as you breathe out, stabilise and go onto tiptoes. Breathe in and lengthen your spine in this position, working the tiny stablisers in your back and tummy to balance yourself. Imagine the ceiling is a magnet so, as you place your heels back down onto the floor as you breathe out, you still feel as if your head is lengthening away, drawing towards the ceiling. Bend your knees directly over your feet as you squat down slightly, taking care not to stick your bottom out. As you breathe in, straighten your legs and return to the starting position.

Squats 8x

Why?

To increase strength and balance in the legs, and mobilise the hips, knees and ankles.

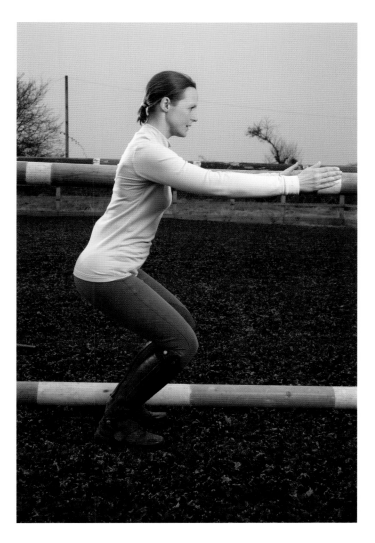

How?

From Standing, breathe in and lengthen throughout the spine, stabilise, and almost brush your thighs with your open palms as your arms swing forwards and upwards to shoulder height, simultaneously bending your knees. Be careful not to stick your bottom out too far, but keep your torso lengthened. As you breathe out, press your feet squarely and evenly into the floor as you straighten your legs and return your arms to the starting position.

Equestrian advantage

Practise squatting down to your own riding leg length to strengthen your position in the saddle – especially useful for eventing and point-to-pointing.

Waist Twist 6x

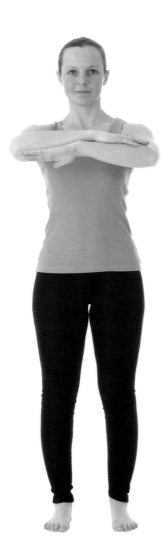

Why?

Strengthens the waist muscles whilst increasing spinal length and mobility.

How?

From Standing, cross your arms in front of you, ensuring your elbows are below your shoulders. (If you hold the arms too high, it increases tension around your neck.) Breathe in as you lengthen your back and stretch your waist upwards, imagining the spine is a bungee then, as you breathe out, twist the upper body, head and neck around to one side. Ensure that your pelvis remains still, squarely facing forwards. Breathe out as your upper body comes back to the starting position, and then prepare to twist around to the opposite side.

Alternative

Try the same exercise from Sitting to better simulate the movement on your horse.

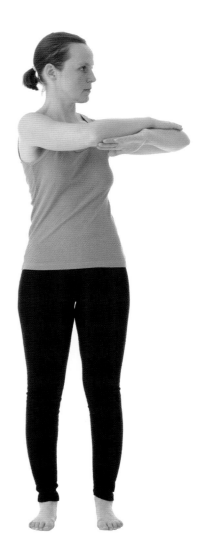

Optional Extra – 6x

Try the same exercise but with both arms out wide.

Equestrian advantage

Helps isolate the hips from the upper torso, so that the upper body can rotate easily around the spine when, for example, asking the horse for travers or shoulder-in, so you do not collapse through the hips or lose balance.

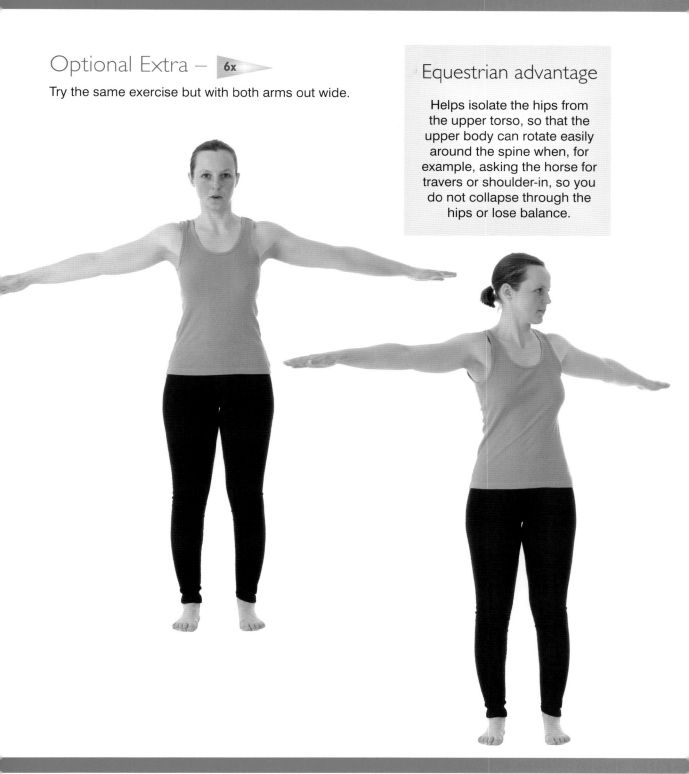

Side Reach 6x

Why?

To lengthen and stabilise the spine sideways.

How?

From Standing, move the toes out, then the heels, then the toes again, until you are standing with legs slightly wider than hip-width. Breathe in as you lengthen your spine upwards and your arm up above your head, stretching your fingers up towards the ceiling or sky, then reach the arm over your head and towards the opposite side of the room or arena, being careful not to fall forwards or back. Your hips should remain still and level, not pushed out or dropping to the side. Enjoy the stretch along the side of your ribcage as you breathe in. Then return on the next out-breath and prepare to bend to the other side.

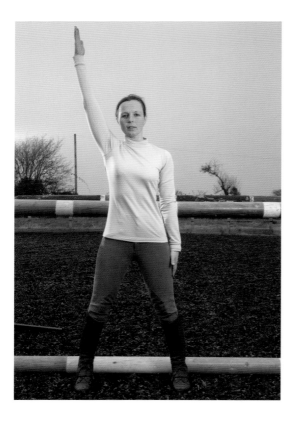
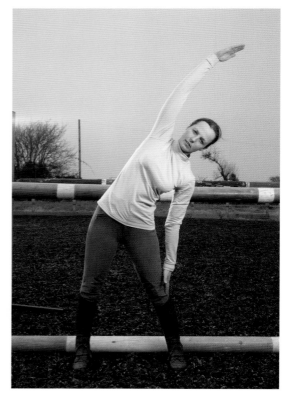

Alternative

Try the same exercise from Sitting, or mounted.

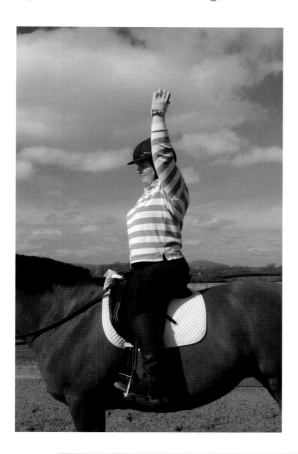
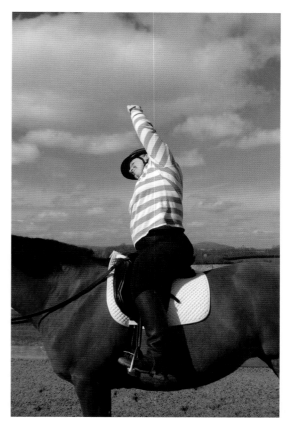

Equestrian advantage

This stretches the quadratus lumborum in the waist, a mobilising muscle. This can often overwork in equestrians and so wrongly takes over the stabilising role of the gluteus medius muscle, if this has become weak, either through ill-use, overuse or injury. Riders can carry a lot of stiffness and tension in this area. Side reach helps to produce a torso that is more independent of the pelvis.

Standing on One Leg 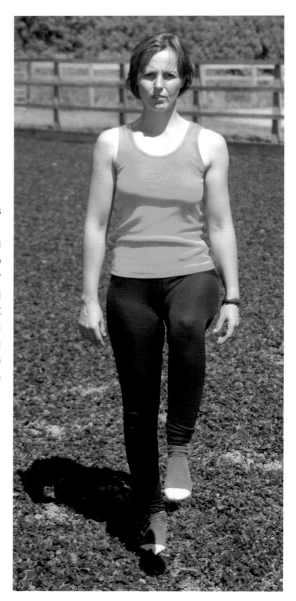 6x

Why?

Centres and strengthens the body, whilst assisting learning to balance from within.

How?

Stand with your pelvis in neutral and legs together, lengthening out from your spine. Breathe in to prepare and stabilise and, as you breathe out, transfer your weight gradually onto one leg as you peel the heel then the toe of your opposite foot off the floor, until you are standing on one leg. Ensure your pelvis is level and not hitched up on one side. Breathe in to lengthen up and feel the tiny stabilising muscles working to keep you upright and level. As you breathe out, carefully replace the foot so as not to disturb your balance – toe first, followed by heel.

Equestrian advantage

A great strengthener for pelvic stability, targeting the gluteus medius muscle in the leg being worked.

Roll Down to Plank to 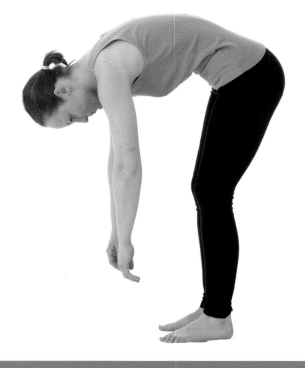 Push-up

Why?

An all-round combination exercise for the body that encompasses spinal segmentation and mobility, challenges upper arm strength, engages the core and incorporates a hamstring stretch.

How?

From Standing hip-width apart and parallel, breathe in as you lengthen up and stabilise, then on your out-breath roll down vertebra by vertebra until your head and arms are hanging loosely.

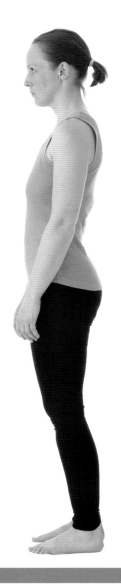

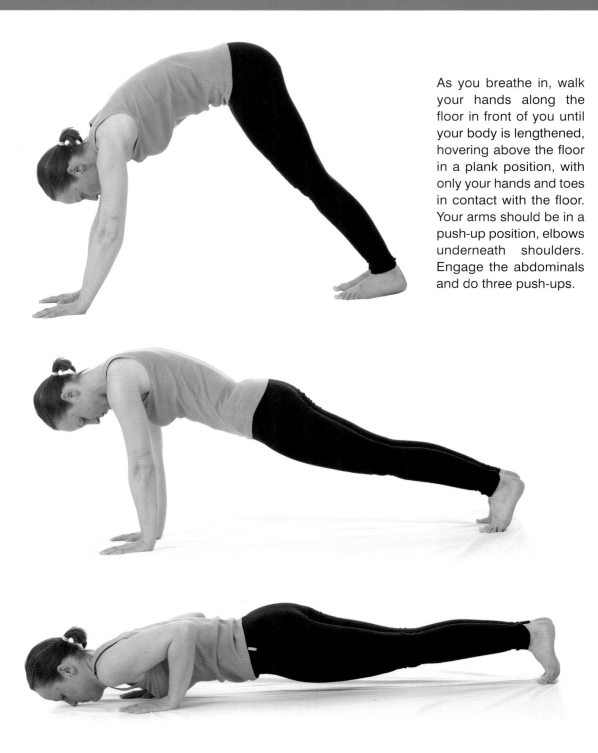

As you breathe in, walk your hands along the floor in front of you until your body is lengthened, hovering above the floor in a plank position, with only your hands and toes in contact with the floor. Your arms should be in a push-up position, elbows underneath shoulders. Engage the abdominals and do three push-ups.

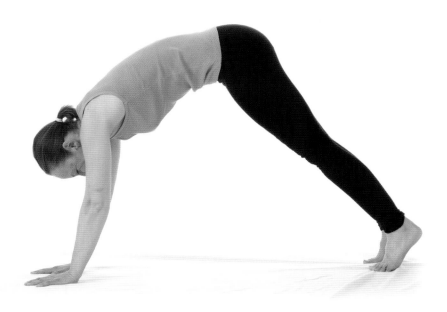

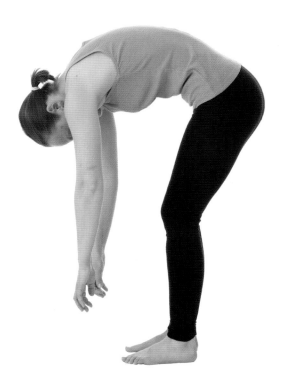

Then start to walk the hands back towards your feet; feel the stretch in your hamstrings as you push back into your heels and come into a pyramid position, with hands and feet on the floor, bottom towards the ceiling. Keep walking the hands back until just your feet are in contact with the floor. Breathe out and re-stack the body, bone by bone, until you are back in the starting position.

Equestrian advantage

A great exercise to have up your sleeve if you're competing and are waiting around between phases.

Exercises from Relaxation Position

Finding Neutral – The Compass

Why?

This exercise is a great starting place for you to gauge just how much range you have in your lower back and pelvis. It also helps you, as a rider, achieve neutral pelvis and spine. A flexible pelvis is essential for riding as it helps you to absorb the movement of the horse. Stability of your pelvis will assist you to maintain an independent seat, plus you will be able to keep your legs quiet and still at the horse's sides as he moves beneath you.

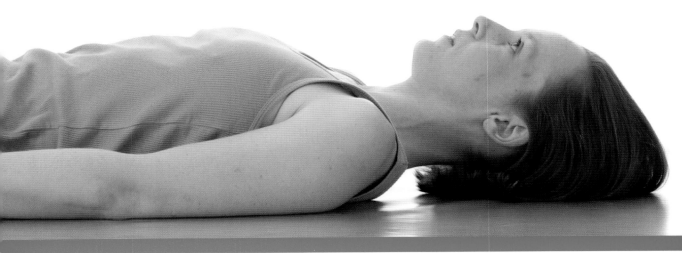

How?

From Relaxation Position, do a simple pelvic tilt forwards and backwards and from side to side. Imagine you have a compass on your tummy with north towards your nose and south towards you toes! East and west are represented by the hip bones.

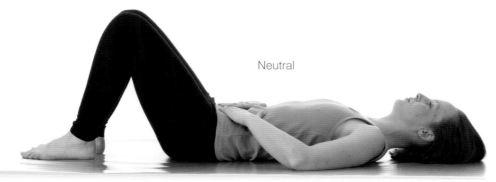

Neutral

Neutral is between the two extremes of the tilt and will be where you feel most comfortable. Find this position for yourself by tilting to the north – you will feel that you have flattened your waist into the ground and you will have lost any natural curves in your back. Gently move your pelvis through neutral in the middle to the south. You will feel that your lower back has arched unnaturally and you will feel as if your tummy is sticking out.

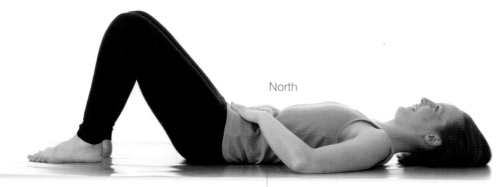

North

waist flattens into mat

Now move your pelvis back through to neutral – imagine your tummy is a table, with a cup of hot cocoa on it. You do not want to spill the drink, so try to ensure that you are not over-tilted to the north or south, or to east and west.

By placing the heels of your hands flat on your hip bones, with your fingers straight, pointing towards one another, you will notice that the backs of your hands are horizontal to the ceiling when you are in neutral.

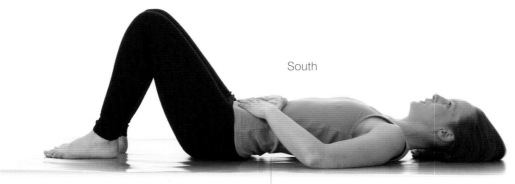

South

lower back my arch

As well as your pelvis being in neutral, the rest of your spine from your pelvis right up to your head must also be in neutral, with the natural curves of the upper spine (thoracic region) and the natural curve at the back of the neck (cervical spine) maintained. Also, you should feel that your ribcage is neither lifted nor squashed into the mat.

Try to memorise this position and practise it so that you can identify this feeling of neutral pelvis and neutral spine, so you can recognise it when mounted.

Optional Extra –

You can also do this from Standing, by placing the small of your back against a wall and tilting your pelvis back and forth. The trick is to be able to do it without disturbing the rest of your body – this should be an independent movement!

Equestrian advantage

The ability to tilt your pelvis is the first step to gaining pelvic stability.

Yes and No Neck Tucks and Rolls ▶ 6x

Why?

To help release tension from your neck.

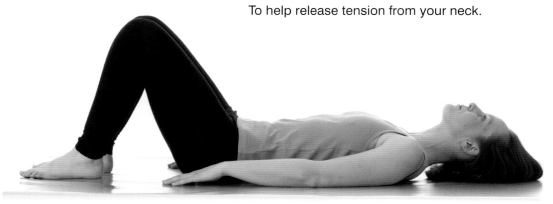

How?

From Relaxation Position, breathe out and gently lengthen along the back of the neck before nodding the chin forward, as if nodding approval, taking care not to force the chin onto the chest. As you breathe in, gently reverse the movement, reaching back with the chin and quietly shortening the back of the neck whilst lengthening along the front of your neck. Repeat six times before moving onto the No Rolls.

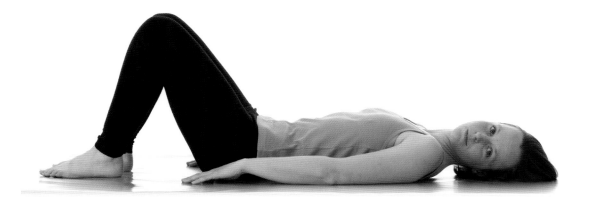

With your head and neck back in neutral, with your focus and face looking up squarely towards the ceiling, start your No Rolls. Breathe out as you roll your head to one side, breathing in to come back to centre, then repeat it to the other side. Do six repetitions, and with each roll or tuck, try to release and relax a little more through the neck.

Equestrian advantage

To help achieve a neutral, natural placement of the head and neck, building awareness of the importance of keeping your focus forward and level. Will help riders whose gaze is often down towards their horse rather than to the front.

Backstroke Swimming 6x ▷

Why?

To build awareness of a neutral pelvis and spine and also challenge upper body stability.

How?

From Relaxation Position, lengthen your body from the top of your head to the tips of your toes as you breathe in wide and deep to the sides of the ribcage. As you breathe out, stabilise your centre before sliding one leg along the mat until it is straight along the floor, at the same time lifting your opposite arm, palms either facing the mat or towards your side/trouser seams (whichever is more comfortable), in a backstroke movement.

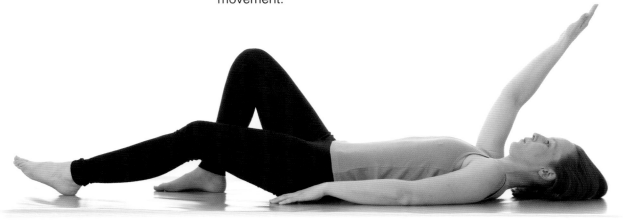

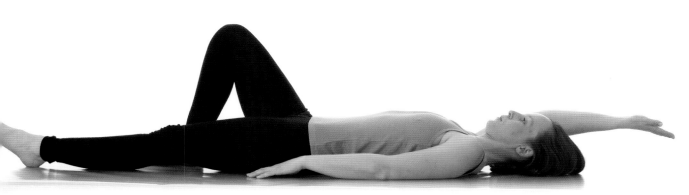

Your hand should hover a hand's width or more off the mat behind you – too far towards the floor and you will feel your ribcage lift and your back arch. Breathe in to lengthen and then return both arm and leg to starting position and repeat with the other limbs. This can also be done with hand weights.

Equestrian advantage

By developing pelvic and upper body stability, you are on the road to developing an independent seat.

Point and Flex
and Ankle Circles 6x

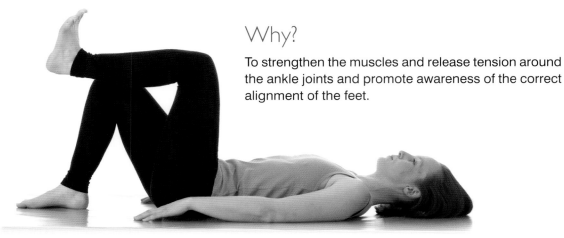

Why?

To strengthen the muscles and release tension around the ankle joints and promote awareness of the correct alignment of the feet.

How?

From Relaxation Position, stabilise as your knee folds one leg up from your hip. To help avoid any tension or gripping in the hip flexor muscles, you can hold behind the back of the thigh. Starting with point and flex, softly point the toes away from you, then flex the foot by pressing through the heel as you then point your toes towards your nose, trying to work through your full range of movement in the ankle joint, but being careful not to over-point or over-flex, which will result in the foot moving inwards sickle-fashion and the toes curling.

Repeat six times each way then start your ankle circles.

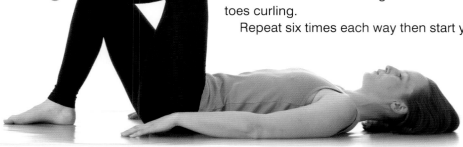

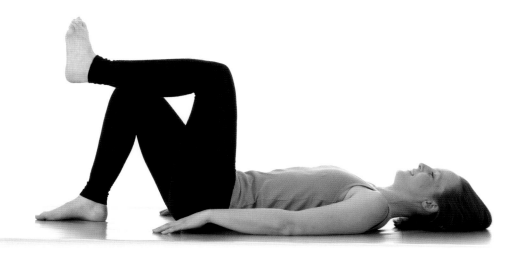

Following point and flex, with legs in the same position, gently circle your foot around six times one way, initiating the movement in the ankle joint. Then repeat the circles the other way, taking care not to curl the toes. If you feel any difficulty or resistance in your ankle when circling your feet, try to work gently on that area to free it up.

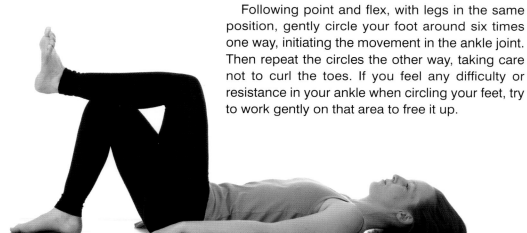

Equestrian advantage

Your foot, being mostly flexed in a heels-down position or in a fixed, straight position whilst in the stirrup, can cause cramping in the calf and stiffness in your foot. Your ankle joints, ligaments and tendons will benefit from the increased mobility and tension relief around the calves that both these exercises offer.

Shoulder Drops 12x ▶

Equestrian advantage

To aid the position of your upper body.

Why?

To open the upper body and release tension.

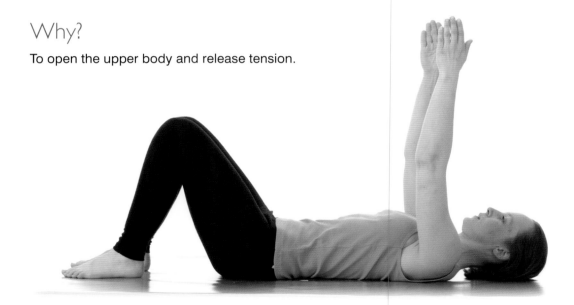

How?

From Relaxation Position, stretch both arms up, shoulder width apart, palms facing each other, fingertips towards the ceiling.

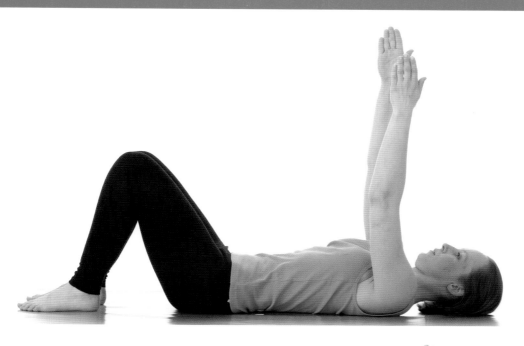

As you breathe in, lengthen one arm up further towards the ceiling, lifting the arm up and stretching out of the shoulder socket.

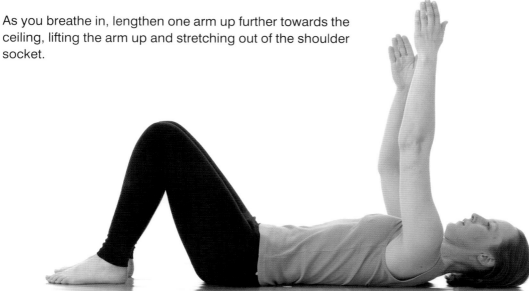

Then as you sigh your breath out, drop that arm back down into the shoulder socket. Alternate arms and repeat twelve times with each.

Tree Hugging 12x ▷

Why?

To open the chest and shoulders, whilst keeping the upper back stable.

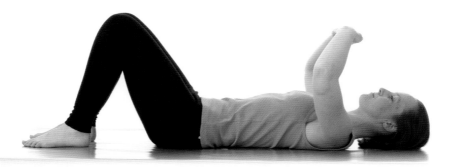

How?

From Relaxation Position, stretch both arms up, shoulder width apart, fingertips towards each other, with elbows slightly bent, as if you are hugging a tree.

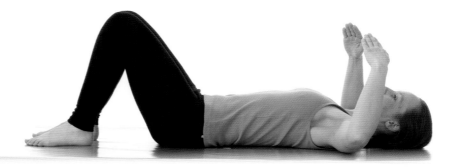

Stabilise through your centre and, as you breathe in, move your arms out to your sides, keeping the elbows slightly bent, hovering a hand's breadth off the mat. Then, as you breathe out, bring your fingertips back together, keeping the 'tree hugging' shape.

This can also be done with hand weights.

> Equestrian advantage
>
> **To aid the position of your upper body.**

Knee Drop and Fold Combo 12x ▷

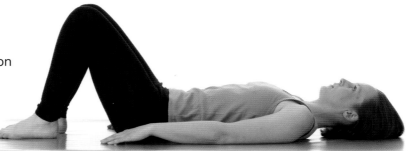

Why?

It challenges co-ordination and pelvic stability.

How?

From Relaxation Position, stabilise and, on the out-breath, fold one leg at the knee whilst, at the same time, dropping the opposite knee out slightly to the side. Take care not to flop the knee out – keep control of it from a stable centre. To fold your knee, imagine you have a rope from your tummy to your thigh and you are encouraging it to fold by using your tummy muscles to lift it up. On your in-breath, return both legs back to the starting position and alternate legs to fold and drop.

Move from a stable centre, so try to keep your pelvis in neutral and avoid hitching your hip or shortening in the waist whilst doing this exercise. Smile!

Equestrian advantage

Co-ordination is a must for riders and this combo challenges the mind as well as the body, whilst keeping you strong and balanced through your centre. Good practice for when your horse makes an awkward jump!

Alternative

Both the above exercises can be performed in isolation, e.g. Single Knee Folds and Single Knee Drops.

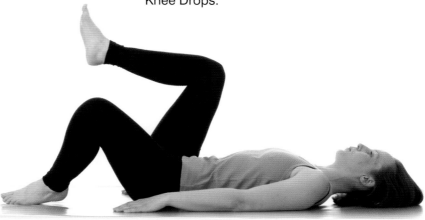

Optional Extra –

Double Knee Folds 8x ▷

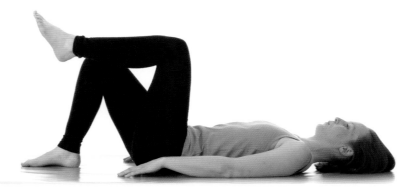

From Relaxation Position, breathe in to prepare and, as you breathe out, stabilise and fold up one leg at the knee towards you, peeling from your heel to your toe. When you have almost balanced it up to its end position of 90 degrees, fold up the other knee to join it. Breathe in and hold that position, feeling your thigh bones heavy in their sockets. On your next out-breath, replace the first leg back down to the mat, toe first followed by heel, then replace the other leg back down.

Take care not to hitch up through your hip when lifting up the second leg; it takes quite a bit of stability through your centre to achieve this without unduly disturbing the pelvis.

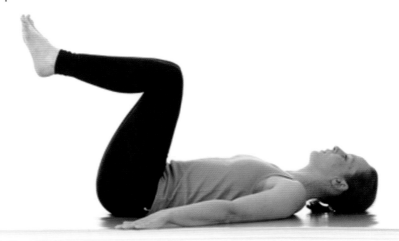

Knee Stirs 6x ▶

Why?

To increase hip mobility whilst improving pelvic stability.

Equestrian advantage

Your first stage in freeing up your hips in order to lengthen your legs! Once perfected, the next stage is Leg Circles.

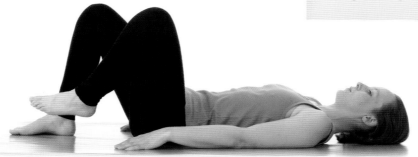

How?

From Relaxation Position, stabilise, then fold up one leg at the knee. Allow the calf and foot to be soft and relaxed down. As you breathe in, circle the thigh bone around in the hip socket, drawing an imaginary circle with the knee on the ceiling. Keep an eye on your pelvis to make sure it remains still and in neutral as you stir your thigh bone around in small circles. Stir inwards towards your body first, then repeat six times in the other direction.

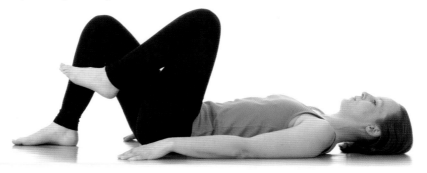

Additional Aid

You can use a folded up stretch band or scarf placed behind the back of the thigh to assist with the stirs to begin with.

Leg Circles 6x ▶

Why?

These challenge core stability through unilateral leg movement as well as mobilising the hip joint and strengthening the leg muscles.

How?

From Relaxation Position, stabilise, then fold up one leg at the knee and straighten it, turning your leg out slightly from the hip. As you breathe in, draw the leg in and up towards the middle of your body then, as you breathe out, circle the leg around and up, back to the starting position. Imagine you are drawing a 'D' shape with your leg.

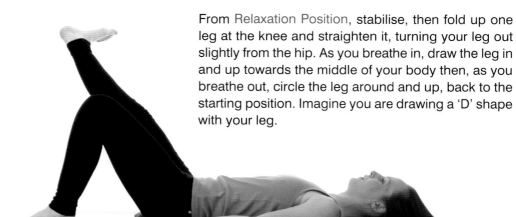

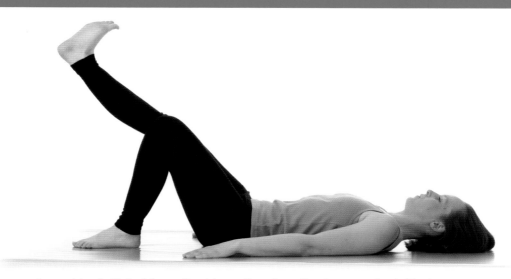

The movement must be initiated from the hip, rather than the knee or foot. Feel that the leg is heavy in the hip socket. Keep the circles small at first until you have mastered the exercise with complete stabilisation through your pelvis.

Repeat six times then reverse the movement before swapping legs.

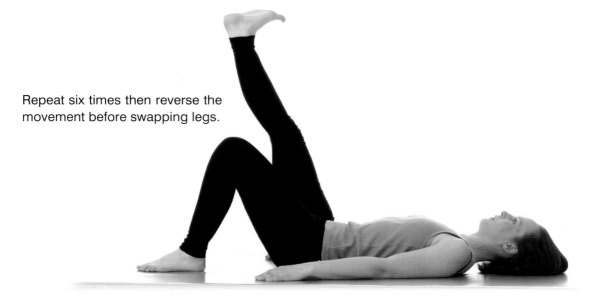

Optional Extra –

The leg that is bent up in Relaxation Position can be lengthened away along the mat.

Additional Aid

You can use a stretch band to assist with the circles. Feel that the leg is heavy in the band so as not to fire up the hip flexor muscles.

Adductor Stretch 20 seconds

Why?

To gently stretch the inner thighs.

> ### Equestrian advantage
>
> Your inner thighs (adductor muscles) are the ones used to help 'put your leg on'. Giving them a stretch the other way will help balance the muscles.

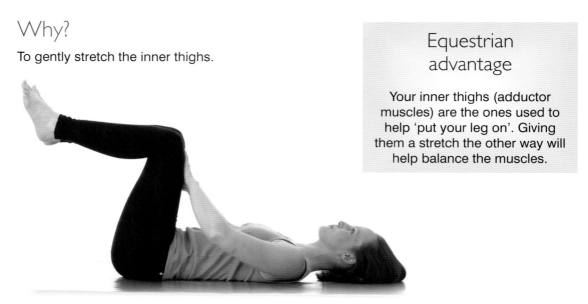

How?

From Relaxation Position, stabilise, and then on your out-breath fold both legs at the knee in towards your chest. Allow width at your collarbones by stretching and lengthening out through your shoulders, then place your hands, fingertips facing each other, onto your knees. Gently part your legs and hold the position for twenty to thirty seconds, allowing the inner thighs to stretch. Then bring the legs back together, stabilise, then return the legs to Relaxation Position with your pelvis in neutral, one leg at a time.

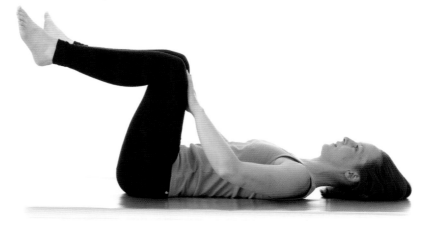

Hip Flexor Stretch `Once each side`

Why?

To open the hip joints by gently stretching the hip flexors.

How?

From Relaxation Position, stabilise then, on your out-breath, fold in one leg from your hip towards you, clasping behind the back of the thigh. (If your back wants to arch, use a stretch band). At the same time, stretch out your other leg along the mat. Hold that stretch for five or six breaths, then swap to the other leg by replacing the bent leg back down to Relaxation Position, then drawing in the straight leg on your next out-breath. Repeat.

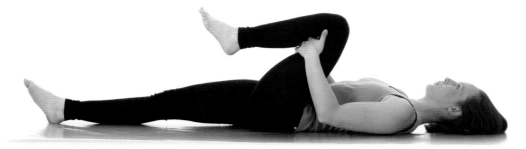

Additional Aid

Use a stretch band if you are struggling to clasp behind the back of the thigh without your back arching.

Equestrian advantage

To stretch the hip flexors (psoas muscles), which can be very tight in riders because of the constant seated position. If tight, this can contribute to the over-hollowing (lordosis) of the lower back which, in turn, will increase backache and stiffness.

Single Leg Stretch 10–20 changes

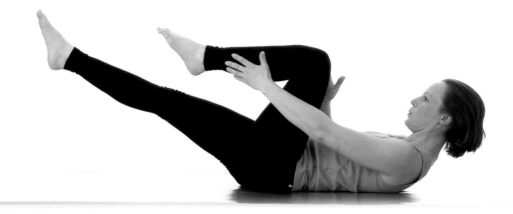

Why?

To strengthen the abdominal muscles and challenge co-ordination.

How?

From Relaxation Position, stabilise then, on your out-breath, fold in one leg at the knee from your hip towards you, followed by the other, and balance them in a double knee-fold, heels lightly connected and knees apart. On your next out-breath, stabilise and curl the upper body off the mat and place your hands on your knees. Take a wide breath into the sides of the ribcage and, on your next out-breath, straighten one leg out and, at the same time, bring the other leg back towards your chest.

Your hands switch to the leg you are bringing in to your chest, one hand on your shin, the other placed lightly on your knee. Alternate between legs, keeping your Curl-up and your centre stabilised and engaged; establish a rhythm with your switches and breathing.

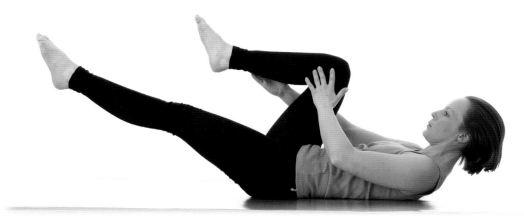

When you have completed ten to twenty changes, fold the legs in towards your chest, then come out of your Curl-up, resting back down on the mat. One at a time, with stability, bring your legs back down to the mat.

Alternative

If you find it difficult to maintain the Curl-up position and remain strong through your centre, build up to it by starting with your upper body down on the mat, and work on patterning your legs and engagement through the centre, increasing your stamina and strength until you can work in a Curl-up position.

Equestrian advantage

This is a great exercise for strengthening your core and stretching and lengthening the legs.

Ribcage Closure 8x ▷

Why?

To build awareness of the effect of arm movement on the position of the ribcage, and to mobilise the shoulders.

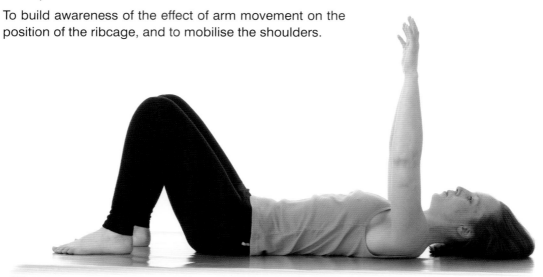

How?

From Relaxation Position, stabilise, then reach up both arms vertically directly above your shoulders, palms facing forwards towards your toes.

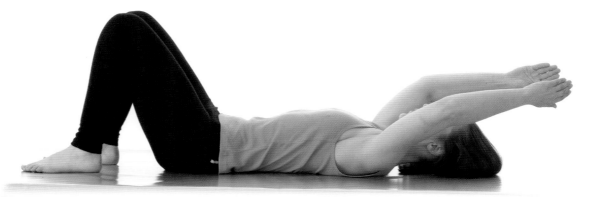

As you breathe out, feel the closure of the ribcage as both arms float behind you and your palms turn inward as your shoulders rotate; feel increased width across your collarbones. Only reach away and down with your arms to the point where you feel comfortable; don't let your ribcage flare or your lower back arch.

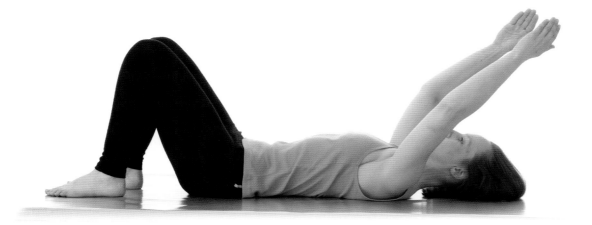

As you breathe in, bring the arms back to the vertical position above your shoulders and on the next out-breath return them to the mat.

Equestrian advantage

A lifted (not flared) ribcage can give instant lift and grace to a rider's position.

Hamstring Stretch 3x each

Why?

To stretch the hamstrings.

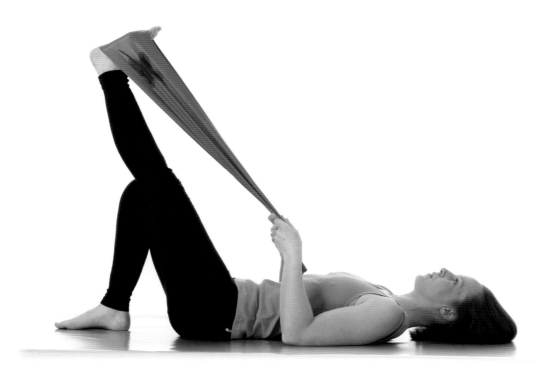

How?

From Relaxation Position, stabilise then, on your out-breath, fold in one leg from your hip towards your chest, casting a flexi-band around your foot. Hold the band so that your palms are facing each other and keep your shoulders wide and collarbones open. On the next out-breath, press your foot away into the band and lift your leg up to an angle of about 45 degrees.

Equestrian advantage

Tight hamstrings are a common complaint among riders – enjoy this stretch at any time, whether you are just about to saddle up in the yard or are between phases at an event and at a loose end in the lorry park.

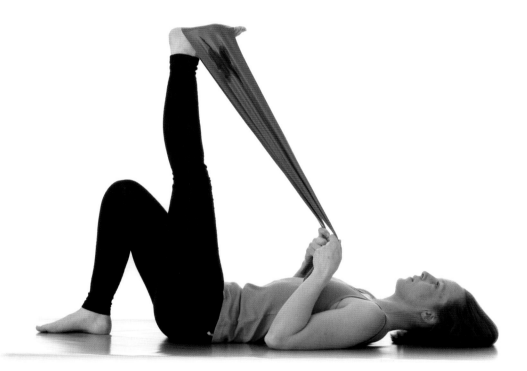

Then gradually bring the leg in towards you, feeling a gentle stretch along the hamstrings at the back of the thigh. Breathe normally and hold the stretch for about twenty seconds. To release, simply bend the knee. If you take the stretch too far it will feel nervy and uncomfortable. Repeat three times with each leg.

Optional Extra –

When reaching the leg up and away in the band, to give the calf muscle a stretch, simply flex the foot.

Spine Curl 8x ▶

Why?

To mobilise the spine, vertebra by vertebra, and strengthen the back, hips, tummy muscles, back of the legs and bottom.

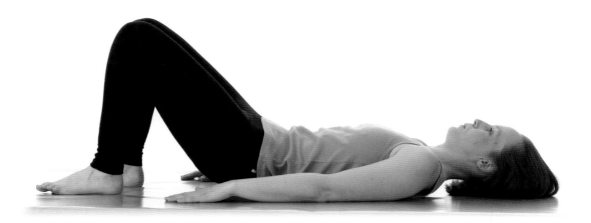

How?

From Relaxation Position, stabilise then, on your out-breath, start to curl the tailbone underneath you as you raise your pelvis off the mat and start to roll up through your spine, vertebra by vertebra, up to shoulder-blade height. Breathe in whilst you feel the lengthening of your spine, then on your out-breath, start to replace the body back down onto the mat, lengthening your pelvis away from you as you do so, softening in your chest and wheeling down through the spine.

Equestrian advantage

A rider's dream! An instant stress and tension reliever as well as a stiffness buster! Helps to develop 'feel' as it pinpoints movement by each individual vertebra the whole length of the back. The exercise can be progressed as core stability and stamina grows.

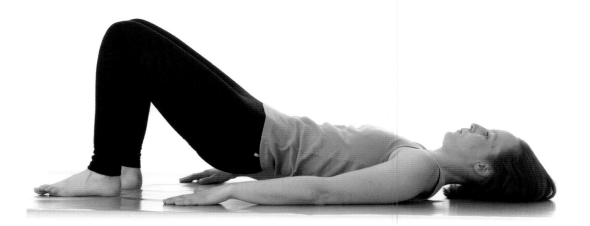

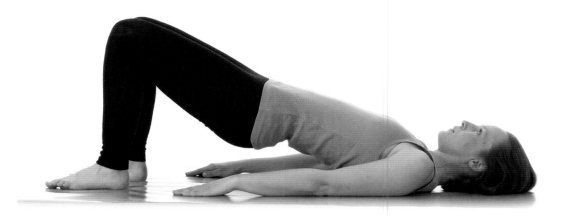

Optional Extra 1 –
Spine Curl with Arms 8x ▶

Why?

By adding the arm movement, you are further challenging your core stability by moving your limbs away from your body, plus it also gives you the opportunity to lengthen and stretch out even further along the length of your spine when your arms are overhead.

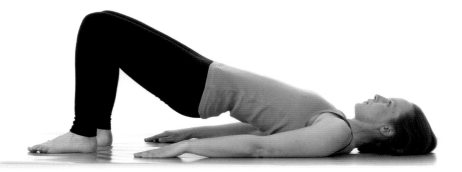

How?

When you are up at shoulder-blade height, on your in-breath float both arms up and overhead, feel the closure of the ribcage and stretch in the spine as both arms reach behind you, feeling increased width across your collarbones.

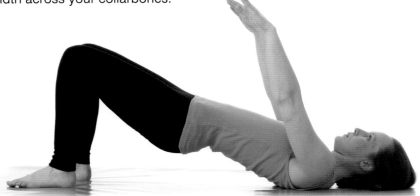

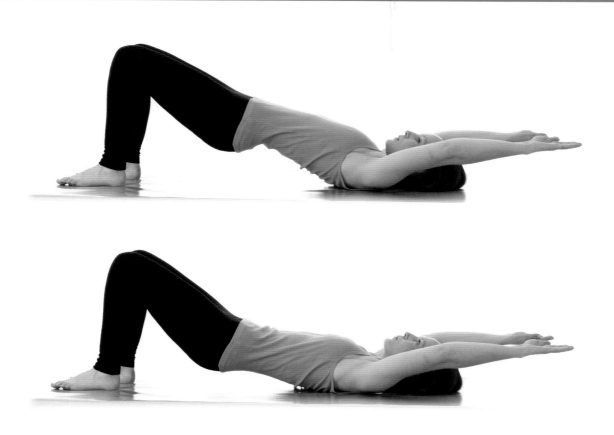

Don't let your ribcage flare or your lower back arch. As you breathe out, roll the body out of Spine Curl bone by bone, leaving your arms behind you, enjoying the lengthening feeling in the spine.

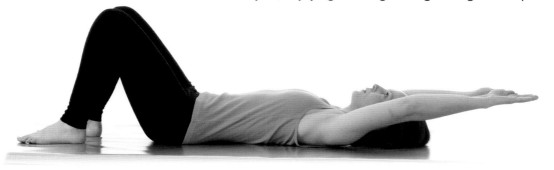

Once your body is back down on the mat, on your in-breath, lift your arms back overhead and down to your sides.

Optional Extra 2 –

Soldier Feet 8x ▷

How?

As in Option 1, when your arms are overhead, stabilise and lift the toes of one foot off the mat and the heel of the opposite foot as if marching on the spot. Do three or four repetitions with each foot before wheeling back down out of your Spine Curl.

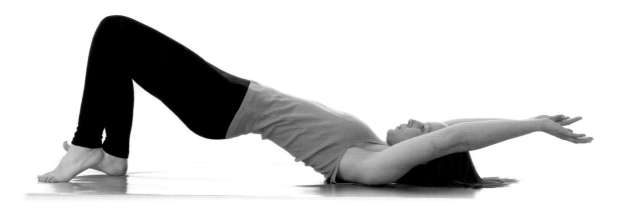

Equestrian advantage

This exercise has the added benefit of strengthening the ankles and the hip extensor muscles.

Optional Extra 3 –
Knee Folds ▶ 8x ▷

> ## Equestrian advantage
>
> An increased challenge that tests core stability, co-ordination and balance; the essentials for any rider.

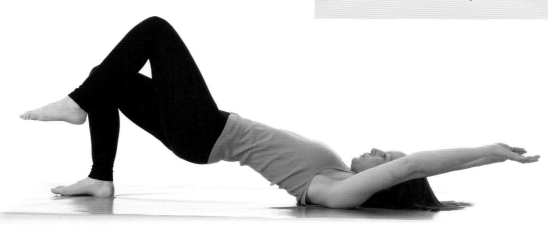

How?

As opposite, when your arms are overhead, stabilise and step your weight into one foot and buttock as you roll through the opposite

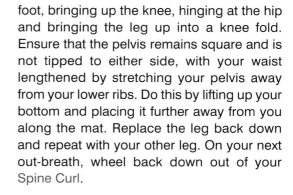

foot, bringing up the knee, hinging at the hip and bringing the leg up into a knee fold. Ensure that the pelvis remains square and is not tipped to either side, with your waist lengthened by stretching your pelvis away from your lower ribs. Do this by lifting up your bottom and placing it further away from you along the mat. Replace the leg back down and repeat with your other leg. On your next out-breath, wheel back down out of your Spine Curl.

Curl-ups 8x ▷

Why?

To strengthen the abdominals.

How?

From Relaxation Position, lightly place your hands behind the back
of your head, fingertips just touching, arms positioned so that you
can just see your elbows out of the corner of your eyes.

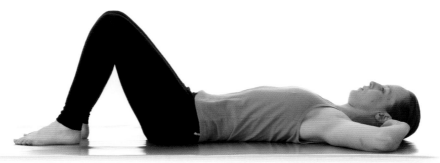

Breathe in and lengthen the back of your neck, stabilise, then on your
out-breath nod your chin, soften your chest and start to curl your
upper body off the floor. As you breathe in, return down to the mat.

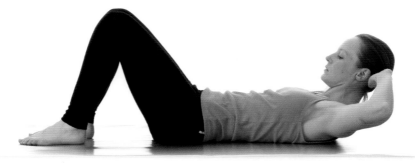

You can further increase the challenge and change the
dynamics of your Curl-ups as your abdominal strength grows
by adding one of the following two progressions.

Optional Extra 1 –

Curl-ups with Leg Extension ▶ 8x

How?

As before, but as you curl, extend one leg away from the knee, returning
it to the mat as you place your upper body back down.

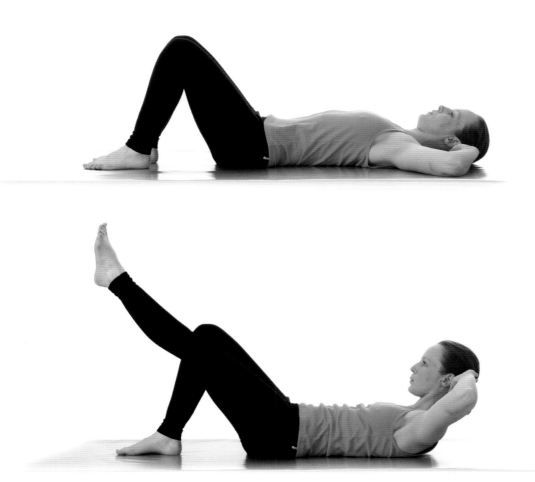

Optional Extra 2 –
Curl-ups with Arms

How?

As before, but as you curl your upper body off the mat, stabilise and, as you breathe in, reach out one arm along your side, followed by the other, then as you breathe out, replace each arm back behind your head, then return to the mat on your in-breath.

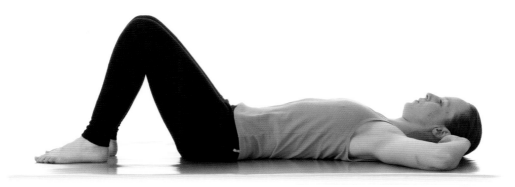

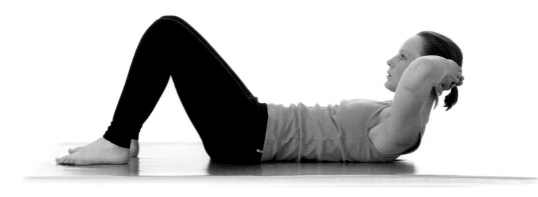

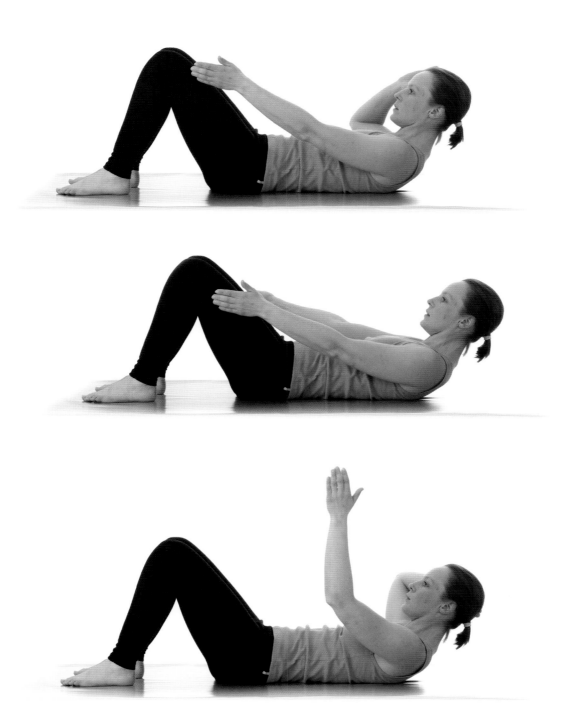

Oblique Curl-ups 8x ▶

Why?

To strengthen the oblique abdominals.

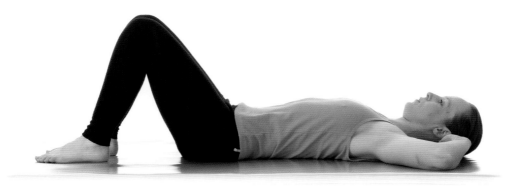

How?

From Relaxation Position, lightly place your hands behind the back of your head, fingertips just touching, arms positioned so that you can just see your elbows out of the corner of your eyes.

Equestrian advantage

The strength through the oblique abdominals assists with twisting and turning your upper body.

Breathe in and lengthen the back of your neck, stabilise then, on your out-breath, nod your chin, soften your chest and start to curl the upper body off the mat, rotating as you lift – imagine taking your ribs across to the opposite hip. As you breathe in, return down to the mat.

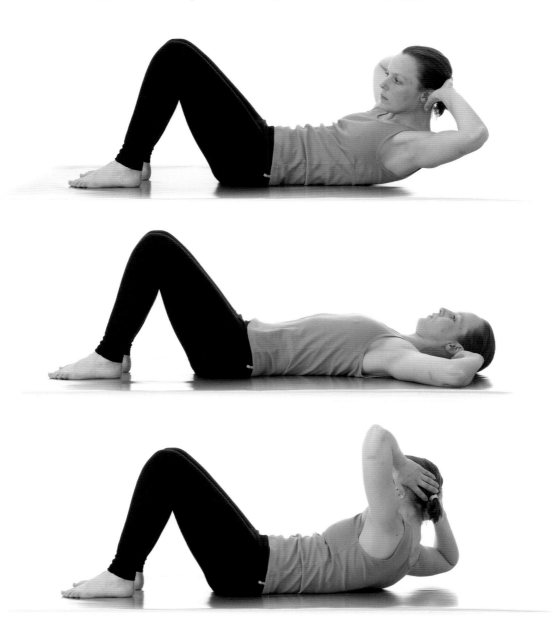

Gluteal and Piriformis Stretch `Once each side`

Why?

To stretch the bottom (gluteals) and piriformis, the muscle that laterally rotates the hip outwards.

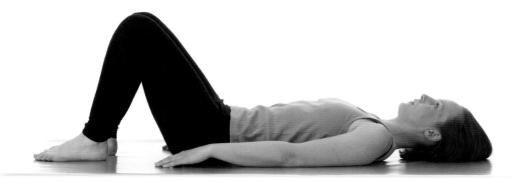

How?

From a stable centre in Relaxation Position, breathe out and fold one knee up, rotate the thigh and place the ankle on the inside of the standing knee.

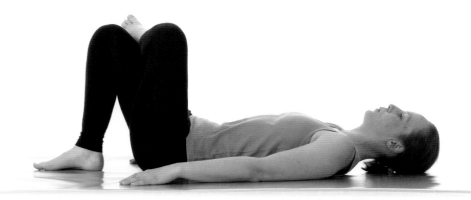

Equestrian advantage

As well as being able to put your leg on with the use of your adductor muscles, it is also essential to be able to rotate the leg from the hip, using the piriformis, and take it off or stretch the leg away and behind the girth to ask for canter, for example.

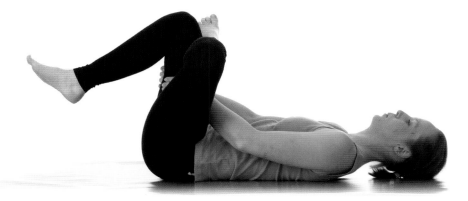

Inhale to maintain the connection, then clasp your hand behind the back of the standing thigh and bring the leg in towards you. Gently press away the other knee with your hand. If you feel tight in this stretch or struggle bringing the thigh forward, use a doubled-up flexi-band around the thigh and draw it in towards you. Hold for about twenty-five seconds.

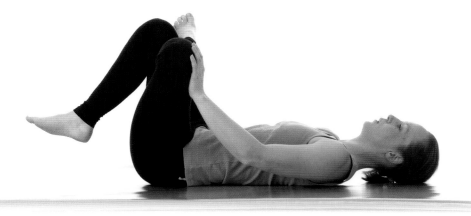

Battement 12x

Why?

To mobilise the hips and move the legs individually in a controlled way, whilst maintaining a stable core.

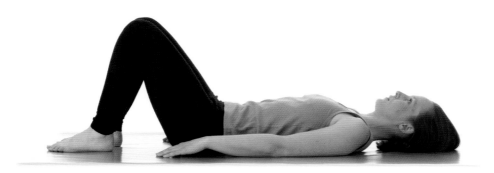

How?

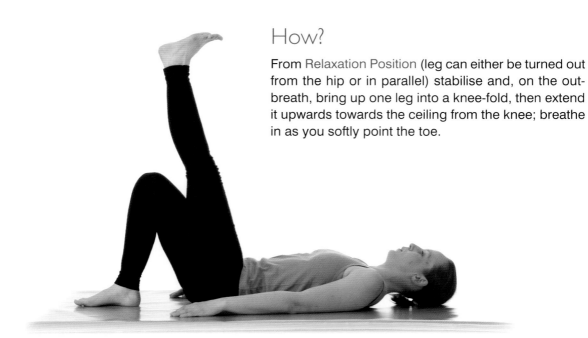

From Relaxation Position (leg can either be turned out from the hip or in parallel) stabilise and, on the out-breath, bring up one leg into a knee-fold, then extend it upwards towards the ceiling from the knee; breathe in as you softly point the toe.

Equestrian advantage

Freedom in the hips allows better movement of the legs and helps develop an independent seat.

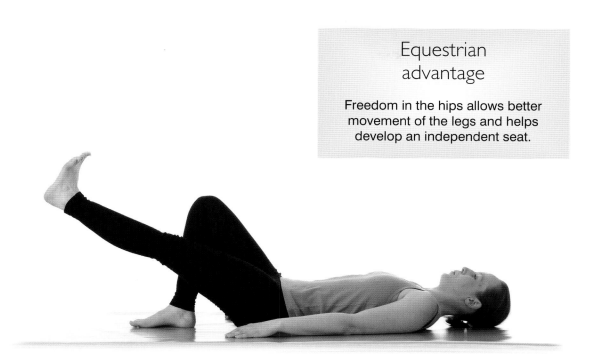

As you breathe out, flex the ankle and lower the leg towards the floor, hovering a hand's width above the mat. Breathe in and repeat the lift and lower, pressing through the heel as you bring the leg down. After twelve repetitions, change to the other leg.

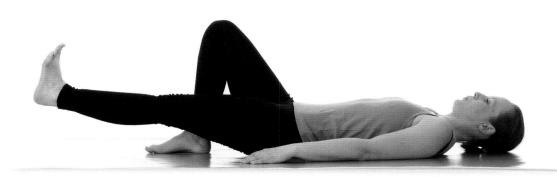

Hip Rolls 6x ▷

Why?

To mobilise your upper body, rotate from a stable core and work the oblique muscles and stretch along the side of the ribcage. With legs up in Double Knee Fold, it is a greater challenge for the core.

How?

From Relaxation Position, place both your feet and knees together, and lay your arms out to the side just below shoulder height, palms facing up or down (whichever is more comfortable)…

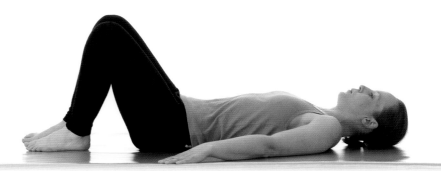

Equestrian advantage

This exercise helps you to free up and move the upper body, rotating through the waist and ribcage to help eliminate any stiffness.

…and, as you breathe out, stabilise and simultaneously roll your head as if saying 'no' in one direction, whilst your knees and thighs roll the other way, still glued together, with ankle stacked on top of ankle.

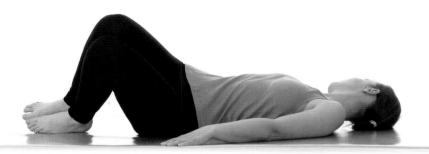

Breathe in to maintain the position and to enjoy the stretch along the side of your ribcage; breathe out to return, bringing back your ribcage first, followed by your waist and then your hips and legs. Repeat to the other side.

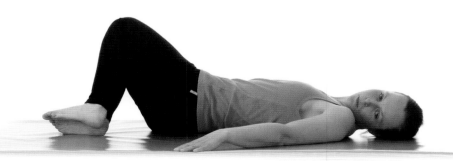

Optional Extra –

Hip Rolls
with Double Knee Fold ▶ 6x

This is a more challenging exercise.

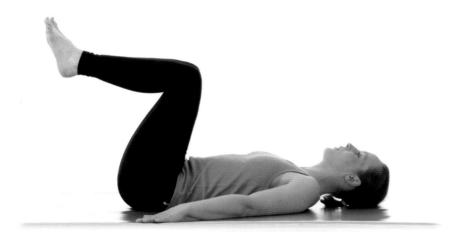

From Relaxation Position stabilise through your centre and fold one knee up at a time into Double Knee Fold and place thighs, calves and ankles together, balancing your legs in this position. Arms are out to your side, palms facing either up or down.

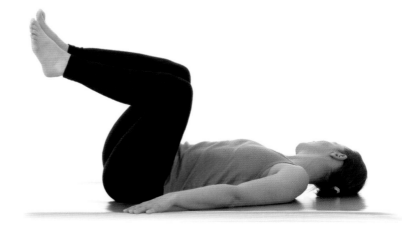

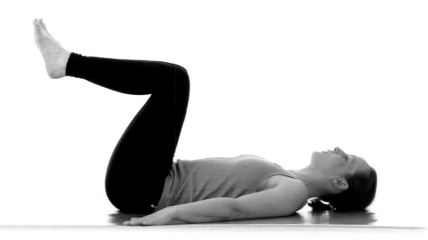

As you breathe out, ensure that you are engaged through your centre before rolling your head one way and legs in the other direction. Do not take the legs too far, because you may become unstable through your centre as the weight of the legs will cause your back to arch. As with the previous version, it is important to feel that you are bringing your ribcage, waist, hips and pelvis back to centre with the engagement of the abdominals, rather than just allowing the weight of the legs to roll in and out.

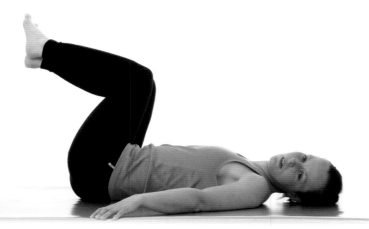

The Hundred

Up to 100 arm beats

Why?

To strengthen the abdominals, stabilise the shoulders and test your stamina.

How?

From Relaxation Position stabilise through your centre and fold one knee up at a time into Double Knee Fold and place your feet together, knees apart, balancing your legs in this position. Arms are along your sides, palms facing down. As you breathe out, ensure that you are stabilised through your centre as you lengthen the back of your neck and curl the upper body off the mat, at the same time lengthening your arms in parallel up to shoulder height.

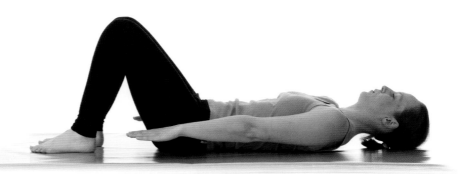

Equestrian advantage

A great warm-up to get the blood pumping, sharpen the senses and release any tension in the upper body.

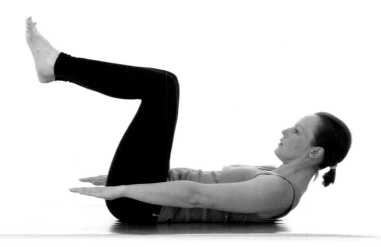

As you breathe in, start to establish a five-beat breathing pattern, moving the arms up and down, taking the hands up to knee height then down to hip height, keeping them long.

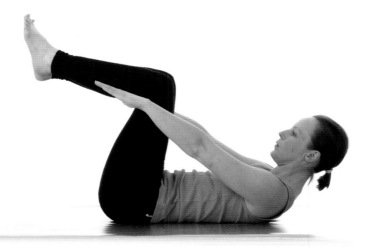

Breathe in one, two, three, four, five, then breathe out one, two, three, four, five, whilst continuously beating your arms up and down.

To come out of the exercise, bring your knees in towards your chest, then curl the upper body down and replace the legs one at a time back to Relaxation Position.

Alternative

Hundred Arm Beat `Up to 100`

To perfect your co-ordination when you first have a go at The Hundred, try it with just the curl-up and arm beats.

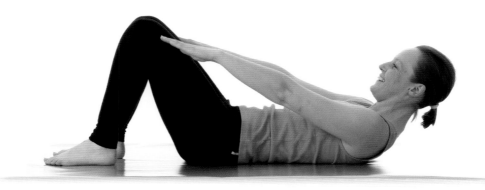

Optional Extra 1 –

The Hundred Plus `Up to 100`

For an additional challenge, you can straighten out your legs in parallel, keeping the inner thighs connected. You can also lower the legs to increase the abdominal challenge – but be sure that your back does not arch. But beware! Much more abdominal strength is needed as you are increasing the weight you need to balance; also, your limbs are further away from your centre.

Optional Extra 2 –
Ultimate Hundred ► Up to 100

For the ultimate in The Hundred, and when you feel comfortable to move on, instead of having your legs parallel, you can turn them out from your hips, into Pilates Stance, with inner thighs gently connected.

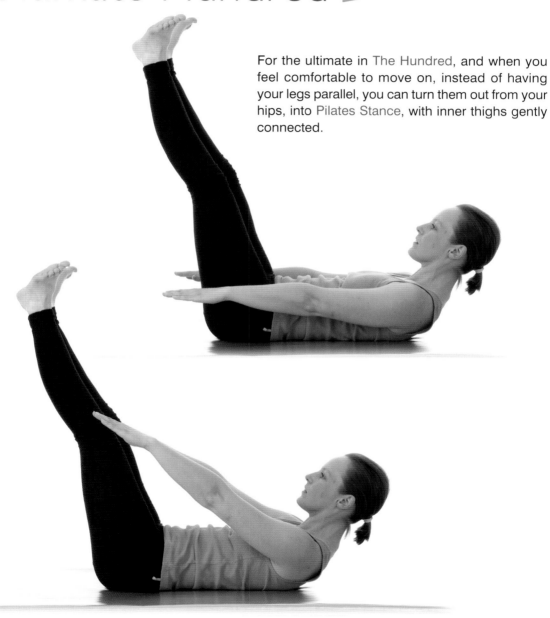

Exercises from Front-lying or Prone

All the following exercises are performed from Front-lying, with your spine and pelvis in neutral.

Diamond Press

Why?

To help lengthen out the spine and open and widen across the collarbones.

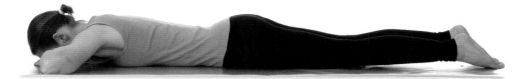

How?

From Front-lying with legs parallel, hands palm-down on the mat, forming a diamond shape, elbows wide. Breathe in and lengthen from the crown of your head to the tips of your toes.

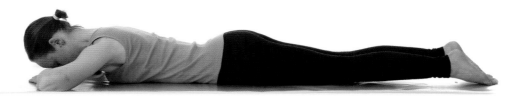

Stabilise and, as you breathe out, lift your head and neck and upper chest off the mat. Feel your shoulder-blades sliding gently down your back as you open your chest and bring it forwards. Breathe in as you lengthen, then return down to the mat, resting on your hands, on the next out-breath.

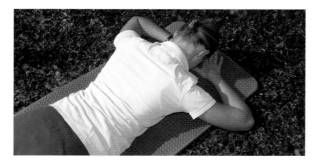
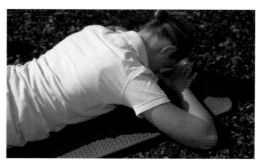

Dart ▶ 8x ▷

Why?

To strengthen the back and lengthen out the spine from the top of the neck right down to the lumbar spine, whilst strengthening the inner thighs, backs of the legs and bottom.

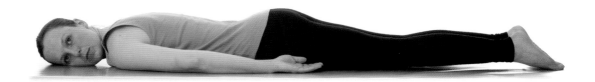

How?

Lie on your front with your face rested on one cheek and your legs parallel, with toes touching and heels dropped out to the sides. Breathe in and lengthen from the crown of your head to the tips of your toes. Stabilise and, as you breathe out, lift and hover your head, neck and upper chest off the floor and gently feel your shoulder-blades relaxing down your back – be careful not to brace here.

Your arms will rotate at your sides, lengthening towards your toes, palms towards your body as they hover off the mat. At the same time, rotate your legs to parallel, heel to heel, connecting your inner thighs. Breathe in as you hold that position, then rest

back down onto the mat on your out-breath, placing your head down on the opposite cheek from which you started.

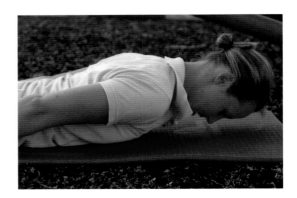

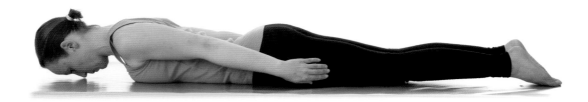

Optional Extra –
Dart with Arms 8x

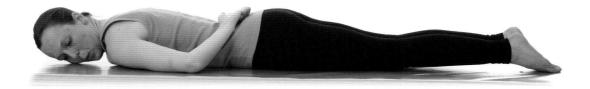

As before, but place your arms behind you, crossed over with palms facing the ceiling and placed hand in hand, resting on your lower back.

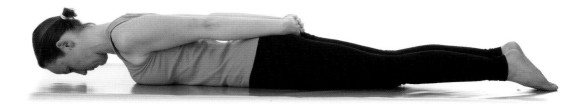

As you raise your upper body off the floor, lengthen your arms and press your hands away from you, along your back, with one hand placed on the other, palms facing towards your head.

Equestrian advantage

A lovely exercise to tune in to the back of the body whilst remaining connected through the centre. Bring that feeling to the arena when you are schooling.

Single Leg Kick 8x ▶

Why?

To stretch and lengthen the front of the thighs (quadriceps muscles), improve
co-ordination, alignment and control, whilst maintaining a strong centre.

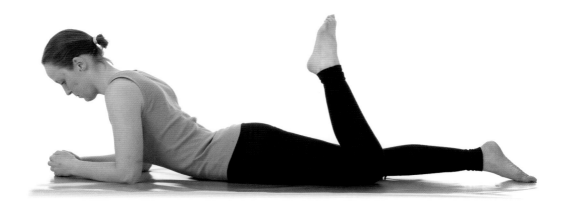

How?

From Front-lying, connect your inner thighs. With elbows bent and positioned
on the mat slightly wider than your shoulders, make a fist with one hand and
clasp it inside the other as you lift the upper body up and forwards. Remain
lengthened from head to toe as you breathe in and open and widen the hips on
the mat, connecting your abdominal muscles from navel through to spine.

From a stable centre, softly point your toe and breathe out as you kick up
one leg towards your bottom, flex your foot as you pulse it once, pressing
through your heel, then point the toe again, lengthen the leg and replace it back
down on the mat on your in-breath. Repeat immediately on your out-breath with
the other leg, making the movements brisk, all the time engaging through your
centre to keep your body stable on the mat.

Baby Cobra 6x

If you feel unable to perform the full Cobra movement (see pages 128-129), you can still experience the feeling of release through your back by starting with the Baby Cobra and then building up to the full version.

For the Baby Cobra, lie on your front with your legs wider than the mat, legs turned out from your hips with your heels dropped out to the sides. Have your forehead rested down on the mat, with your hands palms-down a little wider, at nose height. Your shoulders should feel released and your collarbones wide.

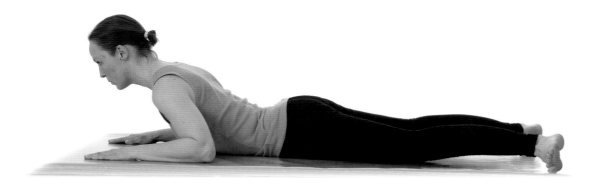

As you breathe out and engage, imagine rolling a marble away with your nose as you start to lift the upper body up and away from the mat, pushing with your forearms, but leaving them grounded on the mat. Breathe in, then on the next out-breath, roll back to the mat, feeling yourself move through each vertebra. It is very important in this exercise to have your core muscles engaged before moving, as this protects your back.

Cobra 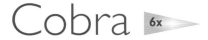 6x

Equestrian advantage

Many day-to-day movements involve flexion, so it is important to balance the body with movements that extend the spine. This is a lovely stretch to relieve aching muscles after a hard day in the saddle.

Why?

To encourage strength and mobility along the back and front of the body, lengthening the spine, opening the chest and hips.

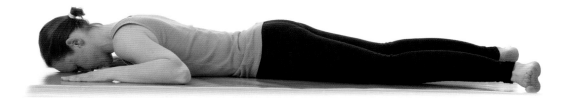

How?

Lie on your front with your legs wider than the mat, legs turned out from your hips with your heels dropped out to the sides. Have your forehead rested down on the mat, with your hands palms down a little wider, at nose height. Your shoulders should feel released and your collarbones wide.

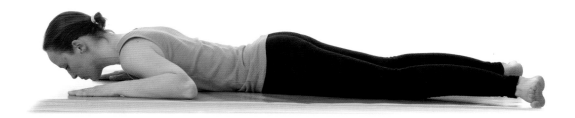

As you breathe out and engage, imagine rolling a marble away with your nose as you start to lift your upper body up and away from the mat, pushing away with the lower arms until they leave the mat and you are balanced on your hands.

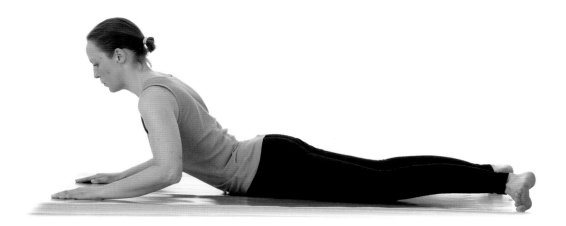

Breathe in then, on the next out-breath, come back to the mat, feeling yourself move through each vertebra. It is essential in this exercise to have your core muscles engaged before moving, as this protects your back.

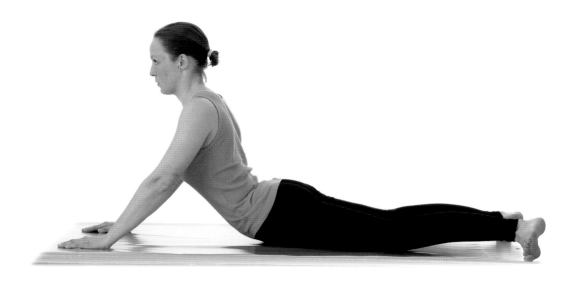

Exercises from Four-point Kneeling

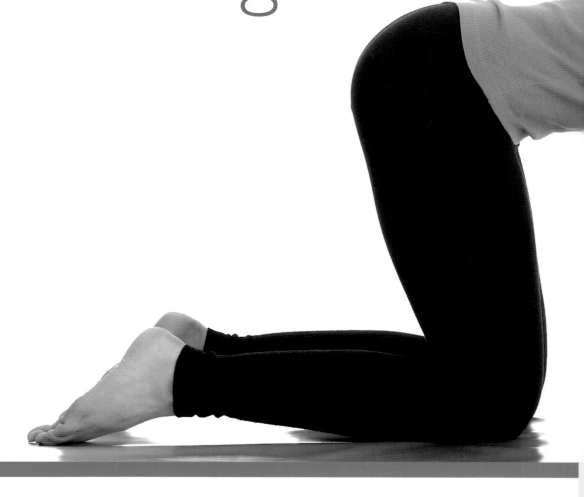

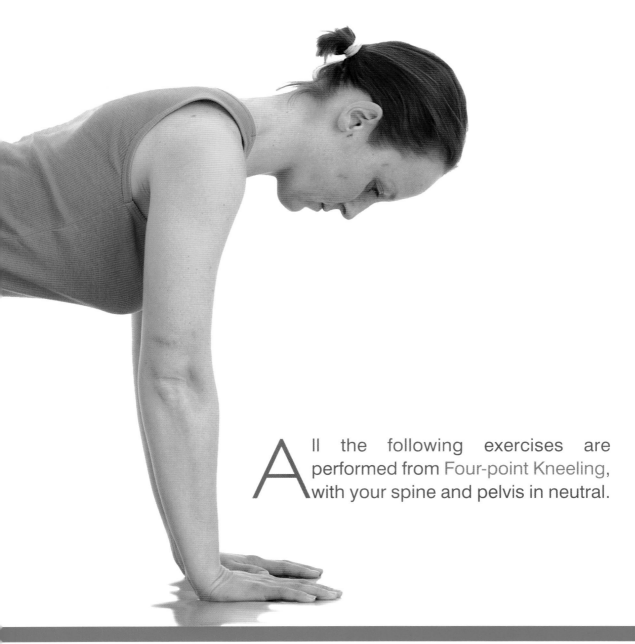

All the following exercises are performed from Four-point Kneeling, with your spine and pelvis in neutral.

Thread the Needle

Why?

To encourage a balanced and controlled rotation of the spine that will aid upper body stability.

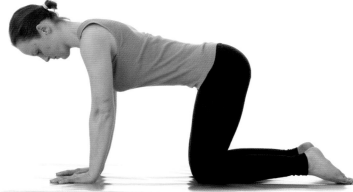

How?

From Four-point Kneeling, breathe in and feel yourself lengthen from the crown of your head through to your seat bones. Stabilise, then, as you breathe out, transfer your weight onto the standing hand and slide your other hand and arm underneath your upright arm.

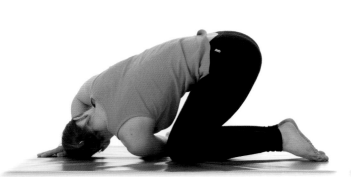

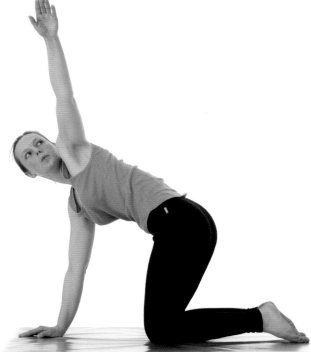

Equestrian advantage

A strong centre is essential when your body goes suddenly off balance, as when following an awkward jump or buck, and you need to recover quickly.

As you rotate your upper body down and sideways, threading your arm under the standing arm; it will bend at the elbow as you continue to rotate under.

Breathe in as you return back to centre and continue past that point of balance and lift the arm up into the air, watching your hand as you rotate it either way, opening up through the chest and shoulders, then return to the starting position and do the same movement with the opposite side.

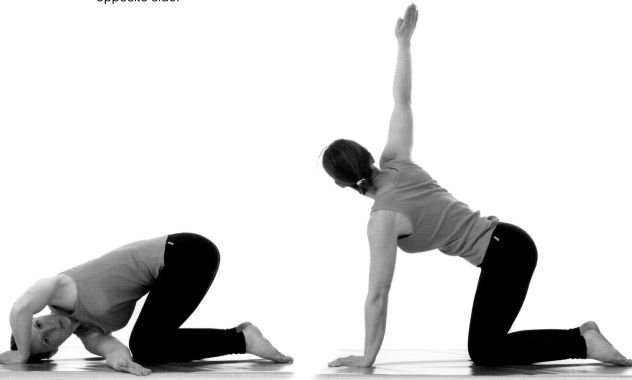

Table Top 6x

Why?

To achieve balance and control.

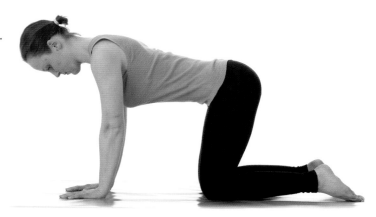

How?

From Four-point Kneeling, breathe in and feel yourself lengthen from the crown of your head through to your seat bones, stabilise and, as you breathe out, take your weight into an opposing hand and leg, whilst you slide the opposite arm and leg away from each other, along the mat, until you are resting lightly on your fingertips and softly pointed toes. Breathe in as you lengthen and balance, using your core, then slide both arm and leg back into the starting position – then prepare to move the opposite limbs.

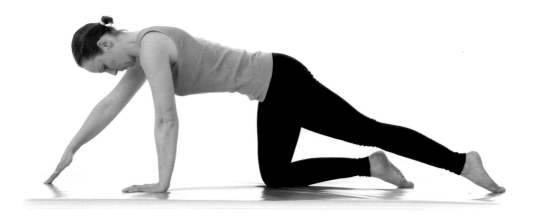

Equestrian advantage

This is great for helping to develop an independent seat! Your centre is stabilised and strong while you are moving your arms and legs away from your point of balance, then returning them with control.

Optional extra

To further increase the challenge, follow the instructions just given, and once both your arm and leg are extended and you are fully stabilised through your centre, lift the opposite arm and leg off the mat, leg balancing up at hip height and arm balanced at shoulder height. Your focus should be down towards the mat. Breathe in as you lengthen from fingertips through to toes, then return both arm and leg to centre.

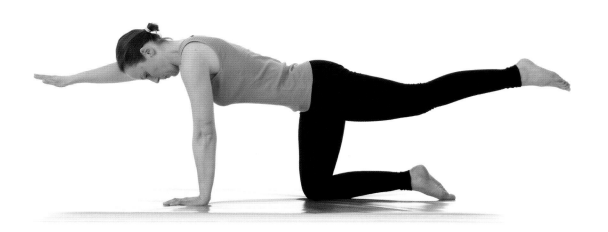

Cat 8x ▷

Why?

To mobilise and release the spine from top to tail.

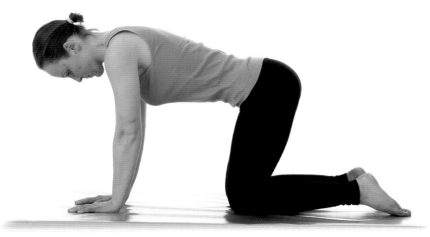

How?

From Four-point Kneeling, breathe in and feel yourself lengthen from the crown of your head through to your seat bones, stabilise and, as you breathe out, roll your pelvis underneath you, as if tucking your tailbone under, and allow your lower back to gradually lift and round, followed gently by your upper back and lastly your head and neck.

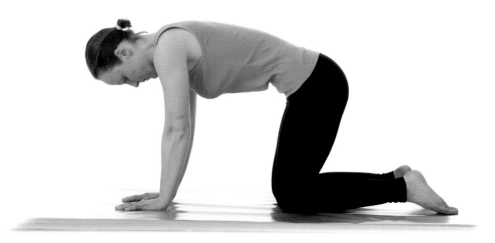

Your entire back will be in a soft 'C' curve. Breathe in as you lengthen in this position then, to unravel, start by rotating your pelvis and upper body back to the neutral, starting position.

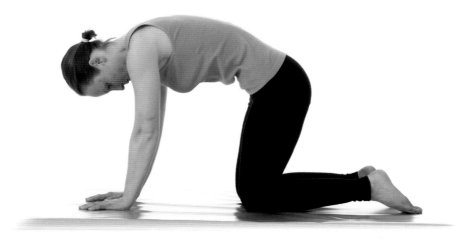

Tip!

Imagine that your spine is an elastic band and, as you lengthen back to neutral, think of sending your head in one direction and your seat bones in the other, stretching your back into neutral.

Equestrian advantage

Fluid movement in the saddle is achieved through having a completely mobile spine, without any stiffness.

Rest Position 1-6x ▷

This stretch is most easily done following an exercise on your tummy or in Four-point Kneeling, as you can either push up into it from Front-lying or sit back into it from Four-point Kneeling.

Why?

To stretch the spine out along the whole length of your body, from your lumbar spine at the base of your back to the top of your neck.

How?

From Four-point Kneeling, breathe in and lengthen, stabilise and, as you breathe out, place your toes together and knees apart as you slowly sit your bottom back towards your heels. Reach your arms forward and relax your upper body down onto your thighs, with your forehead down onto the mat.

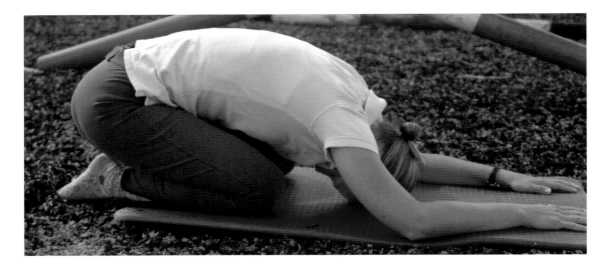

Your arms are lengthened along the mat in front of you. Once there, enjoy the stretch along the length of the spine as you breathe in and gently lengthen the spine on your out-breath, sitting your bottom back even further towards your feet. Sigh your breaths out from your mouth and try to take deeper breaths in through your nose, filling your lungs with air and feeling your ribcage expanding.

Equestrian advantage

Feel yourself unwind after a hard day in the saddle with this enjoyable stretch. You can do this simple stretch after you have run through your Pilates exercises, or just enjoy it alone when you feel a little ragged and want to shut out the rest of the world.

To come out of this stretch, sit your bottom more towards your feet, slide your arms back in towards you and start to re-stack the spine, coming up into kneeling or high kneeling. Allow your head to clear before standing up: first press into one foot, then the other until you are in standing. Enjoy the sensation of relaxation and well-being following this stretch!

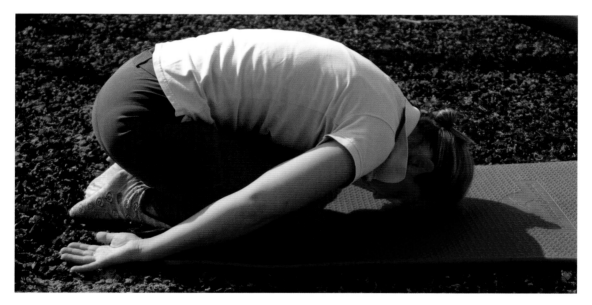

Variation

You can either spread your knees wide and have your feet together, or keep your knees together if you want to stretch out the lower (lumbar) spine. Your arms can either be along your sides or stretched out in front of you, depending on which is more comfortable for your body shape.

Exercises from Side-lying

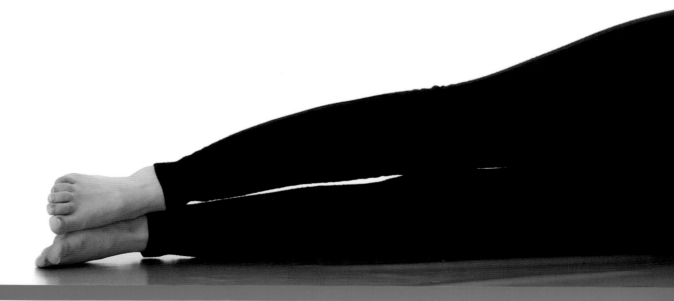

All the following exercises are performed from Side-lying, with your spine and pelvis in neutral. Remember to run through the same exercises on the other side!

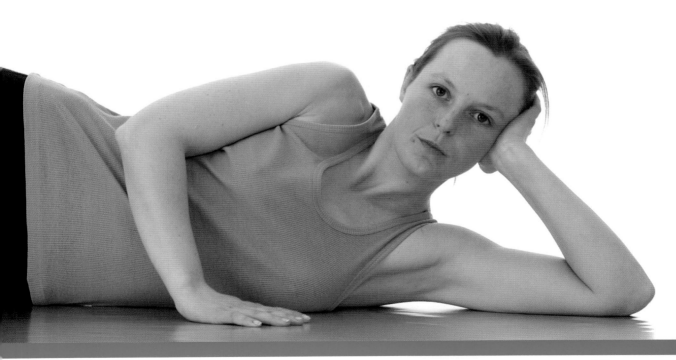

Oyster 12x

Why?

To mobilise your hips and strengthen the muscles around them, whilst challenging the stability of your upper body.

How?

From Side-lying, position yourself with your arm lengthened out underneath you, a pillow placed on top and your head rested down on the pillow.

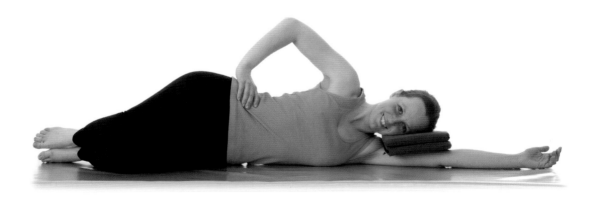

Your hand can be either on your hip, ensuring your hips remain stacked one on top of the other with a long waist, or placed down in front of you. Have your back, bottom and feet in line with the mat and your knees bent and together.

Equestrian advantage

Strong gluteus medius muscles are essential for pelvic stability. Weakness can often be the cause of hip-hitching or crookedness in the saddle.

Stabilise and, as you breathe out, rotate your upper thigh from your hip, pressing forwards and upwards, then return to the starting position on your in-breath.

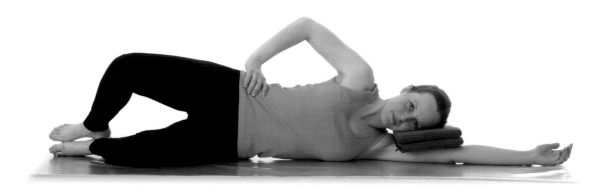

Tip!

Try positioning your legs in your usual riding leg length for maximum 'in the saddle' effect!

Arm Openings 8x ▷

Why?

To open and rotate the upper body, opening through the front of the chest.

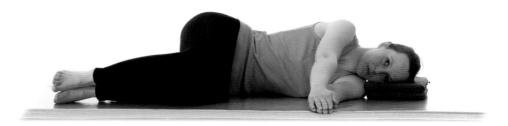

How?

Lie with your legs bent out in front of you from your hip, hip stacked on top of hip, knee on top of knee, with lower legs positioned as if sitting on a chair. Have your arms lengthened out in front of you, palm on top of palm. Have a cushion underneath your head, with three-quarters of it positioned behind you, as you will be rolling your head backwards. Breathe in as you prepare to move, stabilise and then lift the top arm up and move it backwards, rotating your upper body at the same time.

Your knees and pelvis remain still. Follow the position of your palm with your head, and then return to the starting position on your out-breath.

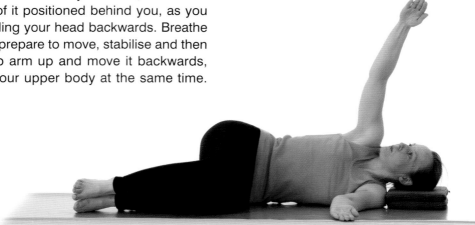

Optional Extra –

Arm Openings with Chest Release 8x

As before, but when you reach the arm out and behind you, take a breath in as you bend the elbow towards the mat and open out through your chest, stretching the pectoral muscles, then return to the starting position on your out-breath.

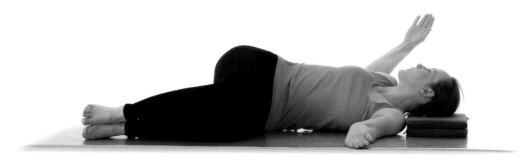

Equestrian advantage

This is another lovely exercise to build openness through the chest and relieve any upper body tension and to practise keeping your pelvis still whilst your upper body rotates around it.

The following leg exercises should be enjoyed as a series together, to maximise their effect. They all target the same muscle groups, from slightly different perspectives, thus they share the same rationale and offer the same equestrian advantages as mentioned under Leg Lifts.

Leg Lifts 12x ▶

Why?

To strengthen the abductor and deep gluteal muscles.

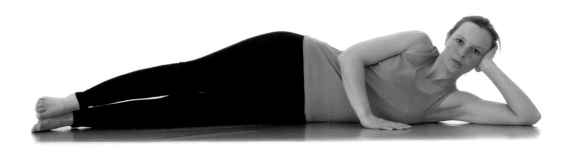

Equestrian advantage

The following series of leg exercises will aid your pelvic and lower back stability, as well as strengthening up the gluteal muscles that will improve your balance in the saddle.

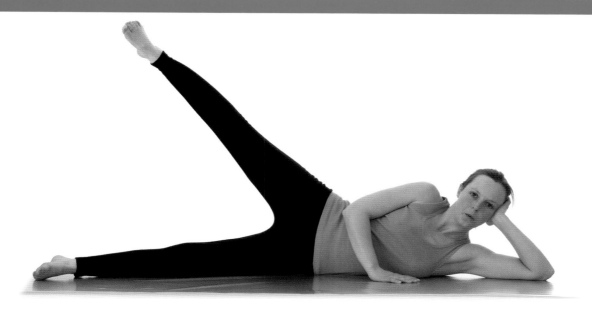

How?

From Side-lying with legs long, one on top of the other, kick your feet forwards slightly so you can see your toes. Breathe in and lengthen then, as you breathe out, stabilise and hover your top leg up at hip height. You can either rest your head down on a large cushion, or prop yourself up on your elbow. As you breathe in, lengthen your leg out from your hip and raise it upwards, pointing your toe then, as you breathe out, push through your heel as you flex your foot, bringing your leg downward to hover at hip height. Repeat.

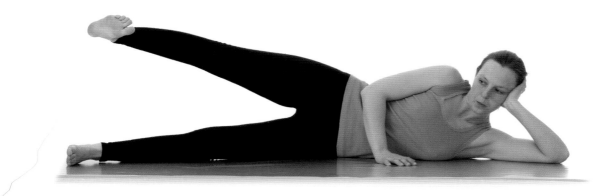

Flex Forward 8x▷

How?

From Side-lying with legs long, one on top of the other, kick your feet forwards slightly so you can see your toes. Breathe in and lengthen, then as you breathe out, stabilise and hover your top leg up at hip height. You can either rest your head down on a large cushion, or prop yourself up on your elbow.

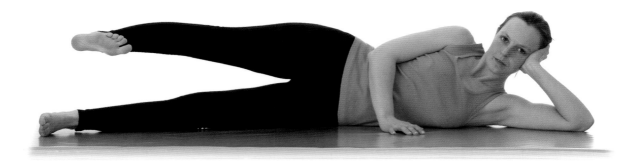

Breathe out as you swing the leg forwards, from your hip, your foot flexed, taking care not to lose your neutral position or wobble through your hip. On your in-breath, pulse your foot further forwards towards your head twice, then swing it back to hip height, hovering above the underlying leg on your out-breath. Repeat without lowering the leg to the mat in between movements. Also try to keep your waist active and long.

Leg Circles 3x each way

How?

From Side-lying with legs long, one on top of the other, kick your feet forwards slightly so you can see your toes. Breathe in and lengthen then, as you breathe out, stabilise and hover your top leg up at hip height. You can either rest your head down on a large cushion, or prop yourself up on your elbow.

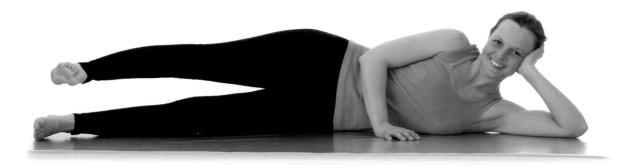

Stretch out through the length of your leg, from your hip, and draw football-sized circles, first one way then the other.

Torpedo 8x ▶

Why?

To improve your balance and co-ordination and strengthen your core, hips and leg muscles.

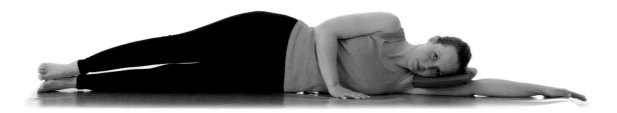

How?

Lie in a straight line, your body stacked and balanced, with your underneath arm out long under your head, which is either resting on your arm or on a small cushion. Place your other hand lightly in front of you to help you balance.

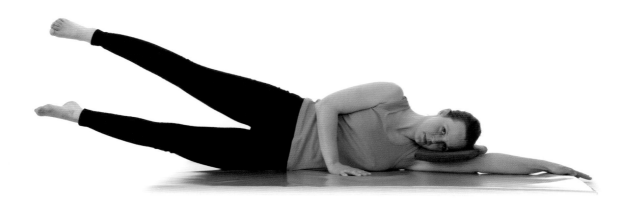

Breathe in to prepare and connect your inner thighs together, stabilise and, as you breathe out, lift both legs off the mat. Breathe in to maintain the lifted position, and then lift the upper leg even further away, keeping strong and connected through your centre. Then, as you breathe out, bring the underneath leg up to join it, keeping the inner thighs connected. On your in-breath, lower both legs together back down to the mat.

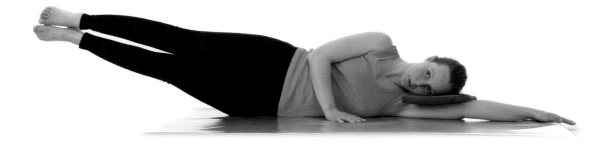

Equestrian
advantage

An all over challenge which really tests your core stability and, once achieved, will be a really valuable exercise to add to your workout.

Inner Thigh Lifts 12x ▷

How?

From Side-lying with legs long, one on top of the other, kick your legs and feet forwards to an angle of about 45 degrees. Bend the upper leg at the knee and place it down in front of you, either resting the knee down on a cushion, or clasping the ankle. If you are able to achieve more length in your waist by not holding your ankle, just place your hand down in front of you. You can either rest your head down on a large cushion, or prop yourself up on your elbow.

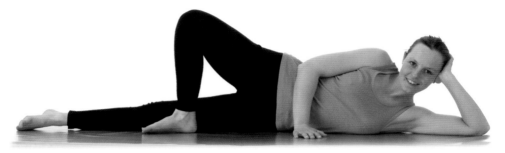

Breathe in and lengthen the lower leg, turning it out from the hip then, as you breathe out, stabilise and lift and lower the leg, with a pointed foot, hovering off the mat in between lifts.

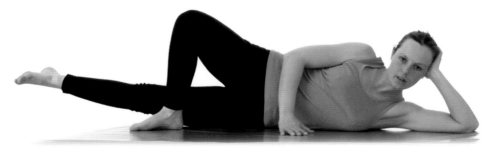

Optional Extra –

Starting position is as above, but instead of having the legs forward at an angle of 45 degrees, keep the leg straight so that you target your adductor muscles too (remember it is the adductor muscles that you use to put your leg on). Don't turn the leg out, and keep your foot flexed.

Exercises from Sitting

As a rider, you may feel uncomfortable or 'grippy' through your hips sitting on the floor, with your legs at 90 degrees to your upper body. To alleviate this, try sitting up on a raised block or a folded mat or large towel, which will open up the angle from your hips to your thighs, plus it will also help you to lift up and out of your waist, thus stretching out your lower back. You can change any of the individual leg positions by substituting them for Long Frog, which is sitting with your knees out to the sides like a frog, with feet connected, which you may find more comfortable.

Studio Stretch with Hamstring Stretch ▶ 6x

Why?

To lengthen the spine and stretch the inner thigh muscles and hamstrings.

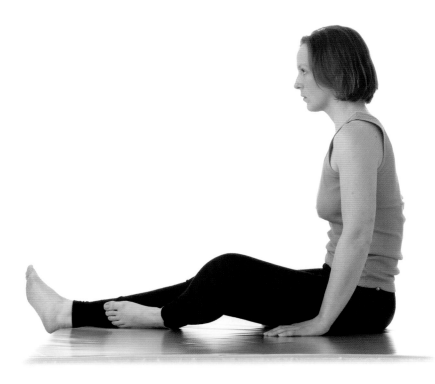

How?

Sitting tall on your seat bones, have one leg outstretched and the other leg with your foot placed on your calf. Your waist is long and your arms are down by your sides, fingertips lightly placed on the mat.

Breathe in to lift and lengthen the spine and, as you breathe out, stabilise and slowly curve your spine forward, bone by bone, keeping your pelvis in neutral. Your fingertips will 'walk' along the floor beside you as you roll your upper body and spine forwards.

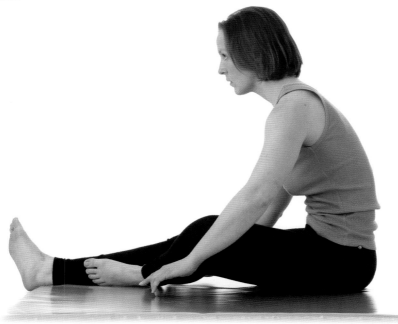

Breathe in to maintain this position and feel the stretch through your spine and upper body, then slowly return to your starting position, rolling through the spine bone by bone.

Equestrian advantage

As well as being a lovely stretch for the lower back and hamstrings, it is a great stress buster.

Alternative
Spine Stretch Forward ▷ 6x

To increase the challenge to the abdominal muscles, try the following from a seated position with arms outstretched, lower than your shoulders, and legs slightly wider than parallel, feet flexed towards you, pelvis in neutral.

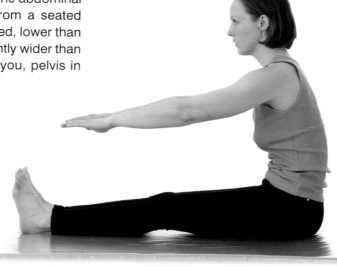

Breathe in to lengthen through your spine then, as you breathe out, stabilise, then nod your head, soften through your breastbone and start to roll your spine forwards, bone by bone.

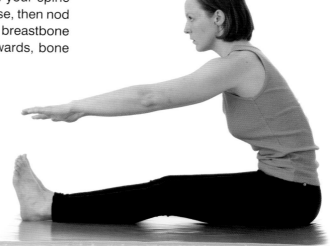

Then, as you breathe out, gently re-stack the spine, bone by bone as you unfurl back to the starting position.

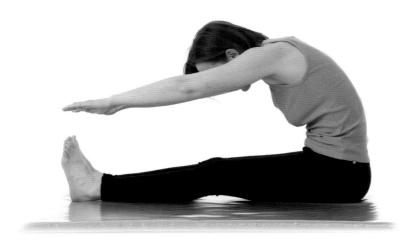

Tip!

Imagine a pepper mill! You twist the top one way and the bottom another. You don't want your spine with its vertebrae and discs to act like a grinding pepper mill and compress on top of one another as you move! Before you move, always think tall on your in-breath and lengthen your spine out from the lumbar area right through to the top of your neck.

The Saw **6x** ▶

Why?

To mobilise the spine in rotation.

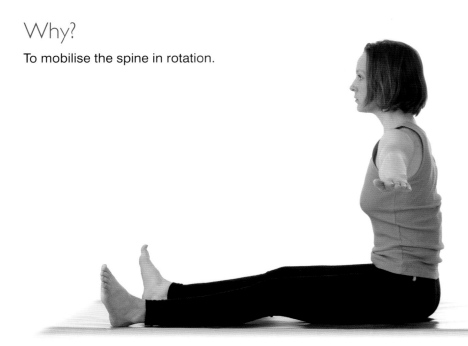

How?

Sitting tall on your seat bones, have both legs outstretched, slightly wider than your mat. Your waist is long and your arms are outstretched by your sides, palms facing down.

Equestrian advantage

This is a great exercise to help with any stiffness in the spine and increase your range of rotation.

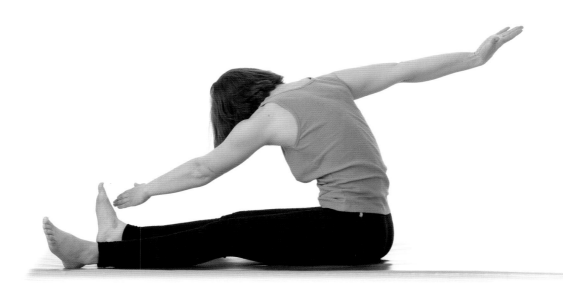

Breathe in to lift and lengthen the spine then, as you breathe out, rotate the upper body around to the side, then flex the body forwards, reaching towards your little toe with your outstretched hand as if to 'saw' it. Pulse your body forwards in this sawing action three times, breathing out. Your head is looking back behind you and your arm reaching away behind your back. Breathe in as you return to centre, lift up as you sit tall, before going to the opposite direction.

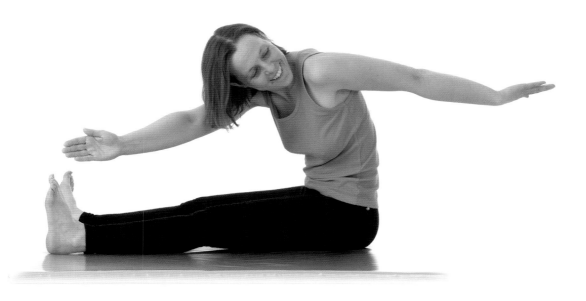

Roll Backs (Halfway) 6x ▶

Why?

To lengthen through the spine and strengthen your abdominal muscles and hips.

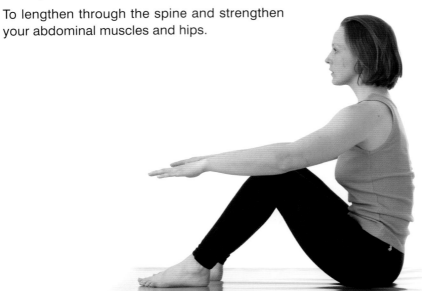

How?

Sitting tall on your seat bones, have both knees bent, feet flat on the floor and hip-width apart. Have your arms outstretched in front of you, slightly lower than your shoulders, palms down.

Equestrian advantage

A lovely exercise to increase your balance and control.

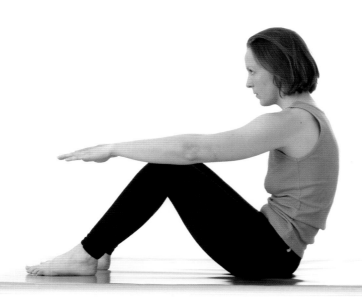

Breathe in to lengthen your spine and, as you breathe out, stabilise, and find your 'C' curve along the length of your back by rolling back through your pelvis. Continue to roll until you are halfway down to the mat, almost to the point of no return. Breathe in and hold this position, then breathe out as you re-stack your spine back up to the starting position.

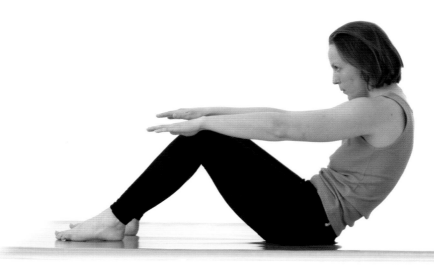

Optional Extra –

Roll Backs with a Band 6x

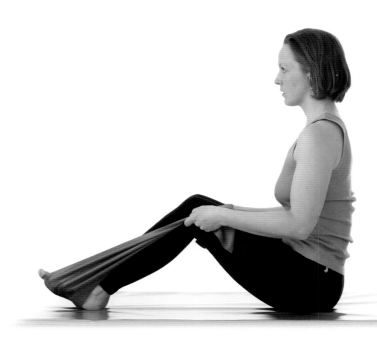

Starting position is as before, but as you roll back in your 'C' curve on your out-breath, move your arms back with you, holding the band along your sides, using your shoulders as if you are sitting up three strides out from a jump, until your upper body is completely rested back onto the mat.

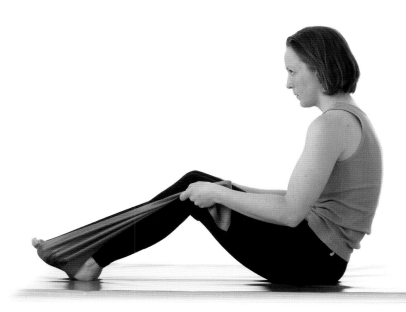

Breathe in to prepare and lengthen then, as you breathe out, nod your head, soften in your breastbone and start to re-stack, using your pelvis to help you go back up to the starting position.

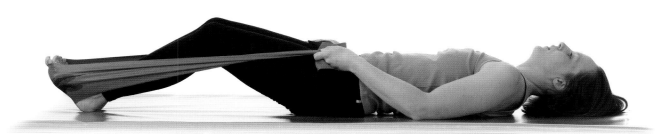

Roll-ups 6x

Why?

To stretch the spine and back muscles whilst challenging the abdominals.

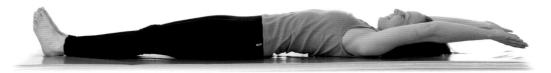

How?

Lie flat on your back with your legs long and touching and your feet flexed. Have your arms overhead but not touching the mat.

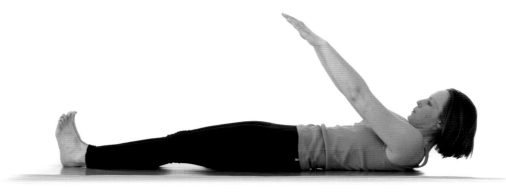

Breathe in to lengthen your spine and start to raise your arms and nod your head forward;

Equestrian advantage

A great exercise to increase flexibility and strength.

stabilise and, as you breathe out, wheel the spine and the body up and forwards, using your pelvis to re-stack and lengthen your upper body over your thighs, with arms reaching forwards.

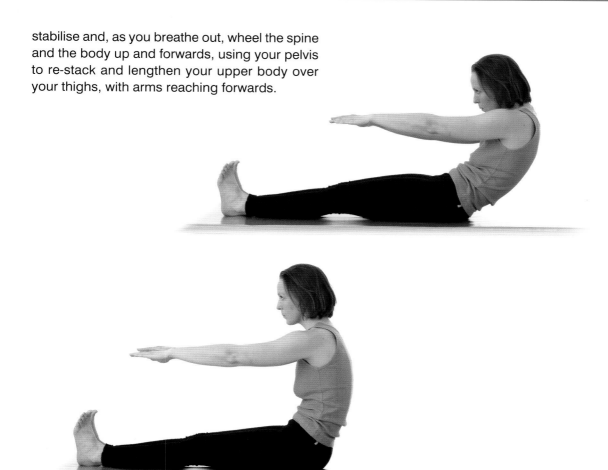

Breathe in as you start to roll the spine back down towards the mat, staying in your 'C' curve; your arms float overhead as you reach the mat.

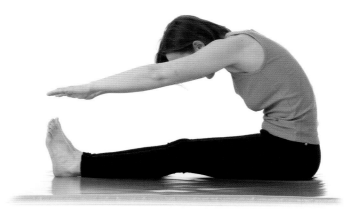

Rolling Like a Ball 8x ▷

Why?

To massage the spine and increase spinal flexibility, whilst working the abdominal muscles.

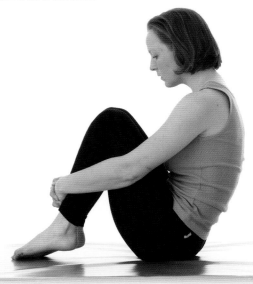

How?

Sit up tall on your seat bones, with knees bent, then grasp your ankles or just above and lift your feet just off the mat, then curl your tailbone under to find your 'C' curve.

Equestrian advantage

A great stress and tension buster! Whilst challenging your balance, working in a 'C' curve helps to mobilise the pelvis.

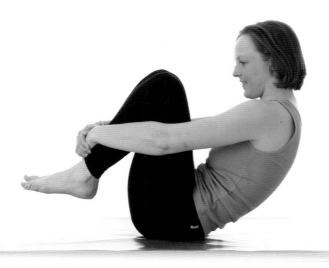

Balance briefly in this position and then, as you breathe in, roll back onto your upper body to shoulder-blade height, where you balance for a second before rolling back to the starting position. Smile!

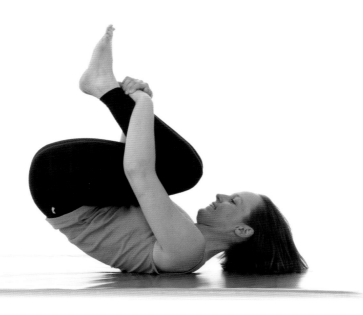

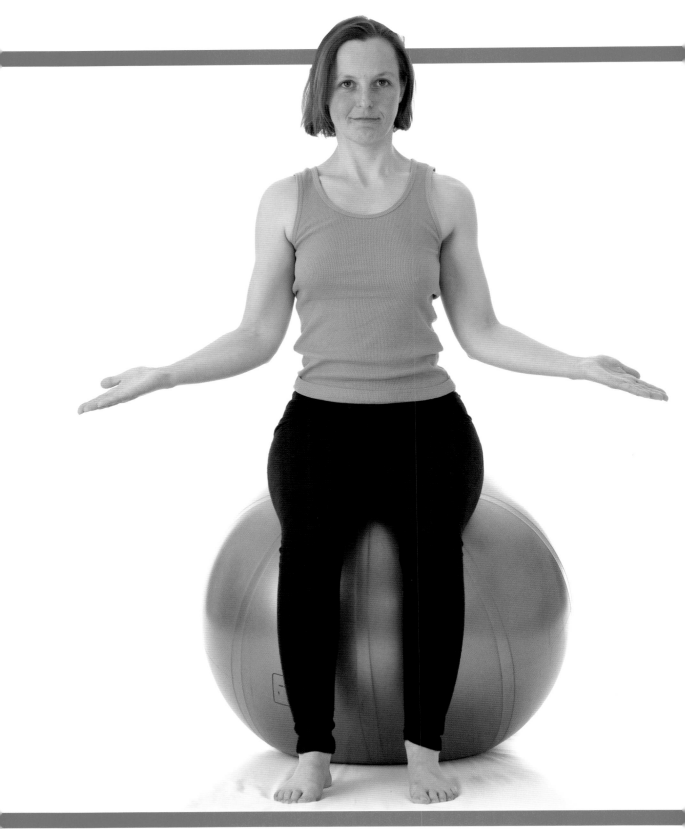

Using the Physio Ball

The physio ball is a great tool for riders as it provides an unstable surface, just like how an unbroken three-year-old can feel! Its instability helps you to strengthen your deep stabilising muscles to help improve your balance and build your core muscles. Even just by sitting square on the ball and balancing with your feet on the floor, you are exercising your deep postural muscles.

When looking for a ball, it is important to make sure you get the right size for your height. Ideally, when you sit on it, your hips should be higher than your knees.

Exercises to try include Pelvic Tilts and Rolls, Waist Twist, Knee Folds, Dumb Waiter, Lumbar Stretch and Diamond Press, but you can adapt many more exercises from the Pilates for Equestrians programme.

Pelvic Tilts and Rolls

Challenge your stability by tilting your pelvis over to the left and right and then forwards and back, allowing your pelvis to roll in and out of neutral. This will help you to free up your lower spine and develop your pelvic stability.

Sitting upright and central on the ball, your back lengthening up, stabilise and hold.

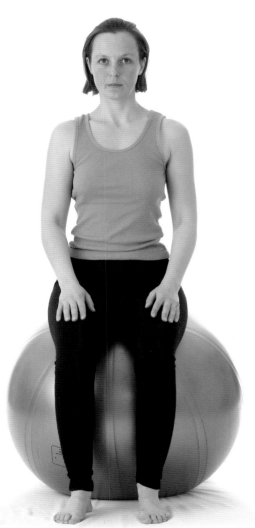

From your upright position, tilt your pelvis over to the left.

From your upright position, tilt your pelvis over to the right.

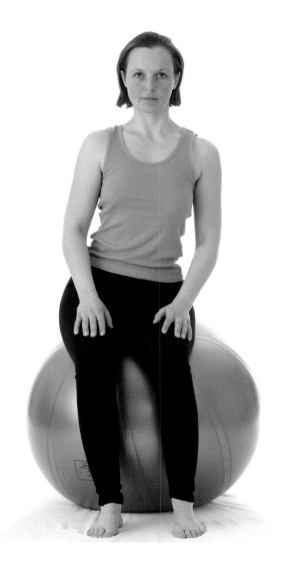 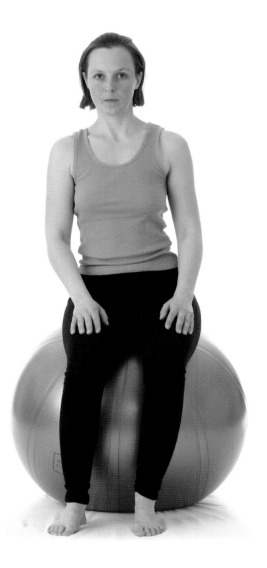

Dumb Waiter

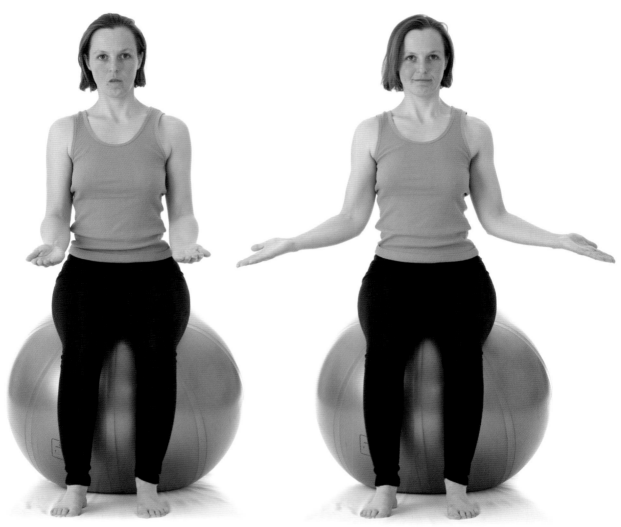

From sitting, lengthen up through your spine and open your arms out in front of you with palms open, elbows under shoulders, as if carrying a just-cleaned bridle. Your elbows are by your sides, but not forced or bracing. Stabilise.

As you breathe in and lengthen through your spine, open your arms out to the side, feeling the movement start and rotate from your shoulders, not your elbows. As you breathe out, return to the starting position.

Knee Folds

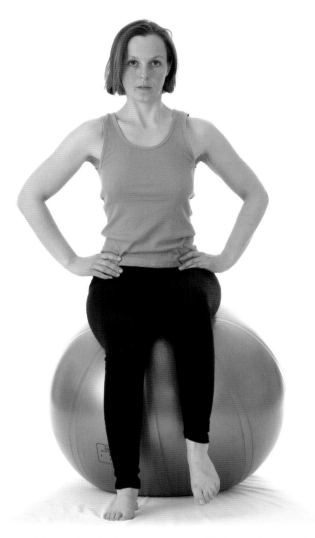

From a stable centre, balance your weight through your standing leg, roll through your foot and fold up your knee, taking care not to drop or hitch up the hip, keeping your pelvis square. Balance in that position for one breath, then replace, with control, back to the floor.

Lumbar Stretch

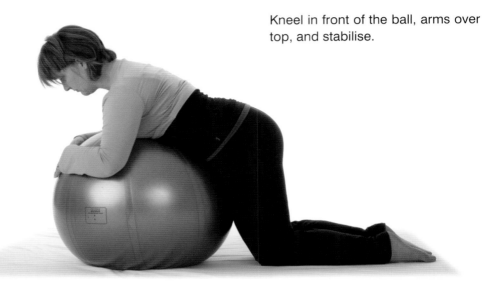

Kneel in front of the ball, arms over top, and stabilise.

Push up with your thighs and simultaneously roll the ball away with control, until your lumbar back is topmost on the ball and your toes and hands are on the floor. Hold the stretch for a breath and then roll back to the starting position.

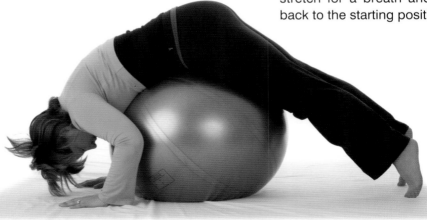

Diamond Press

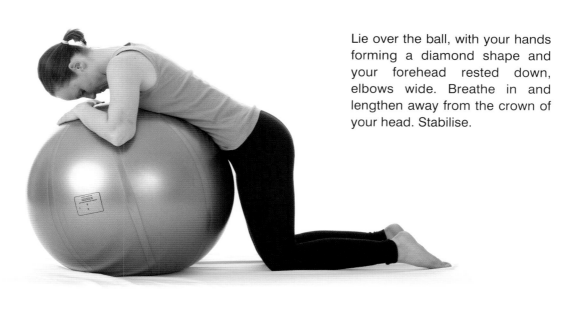

Lie over the ball, with your hands forming a diamond shape and your forehead rested down, elbows wide. Breathe in and lengthen away from the crown of your head. Stabilise.

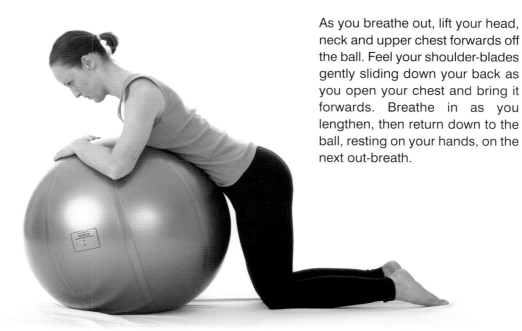

As you breathe out, lift your head, neck and upper chest forwards off the ball. Feel your shoulder-blades gently sliding down your back as you open your chest and bring it forwards. Breathe in as you lengthen, then return down to the ball, resting on your hands, on the next out-breath.

PART THREE

THE HORSE/RIDER PARTNERSHIP

Dianne Breeze 2010

Your
Equine Partner

Riding is the only major sport where the human body, by sitting astride, actually influences and controls another living creature – the horse. By nature horses, like us, are not symmetrical; they can favour one side or the other. Also, they suffer similar injuries such as weak muscles and strains – and they have off- and on-days!

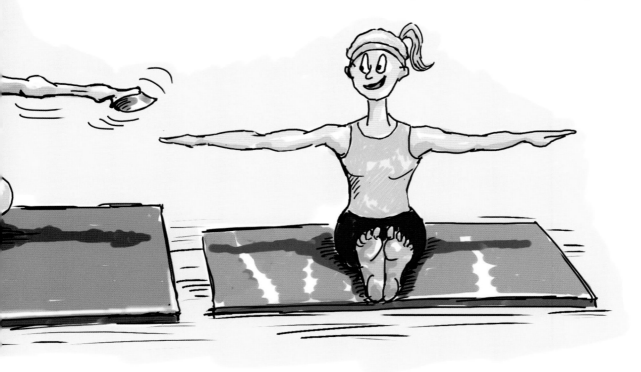

One factor is certain – the horse will adapt his way of going to suit his rider, very often to the detriment of himself and the overall performance. If a rider influences a horse negatively, then a good horse can very quickly slip into bad habits and not perform at his best.

If you ride a big-moving horse, you as his rider may find that you suffer from more aches and pains than you would if you sat on a quieter-moving horse.

One very important point relates to the horse's mouth – the most sensitive part of his body. It is very important that the rider establishes a secure and balanced position, so that there are no undue influences on the horse's mouth and, for the same reason, the rider must remain calm and settled, so that the horse is calm and settled.

Checklist

Once mounted, do a quick check to ensure that your spine is in line with your horse's! It may sound obvious, but how many times have you seen a crooked rider in the show ring? Often, this is to do with the fit of the saddle, the shape of the horse or uneven stirrup length, but it can also be because a rider is collapsing on one side, either because of tight muscles, stiffness or injury. How will you or your horse perform at your best if you are both handicapped from the start? Many of the causes are preventable or, once established, curable. Ask a friend to look from behind.

If you tend always to do the same warm-up routine, try varying it so that both you and your horse vary which muscles you use – and

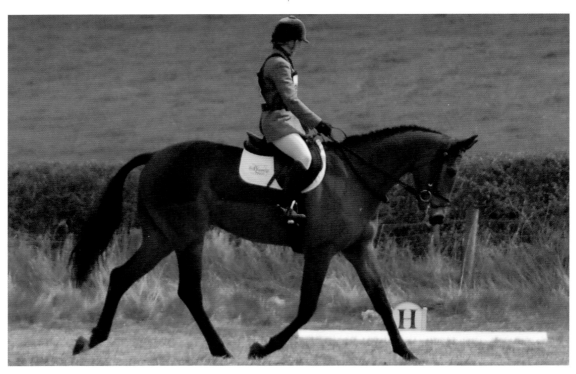

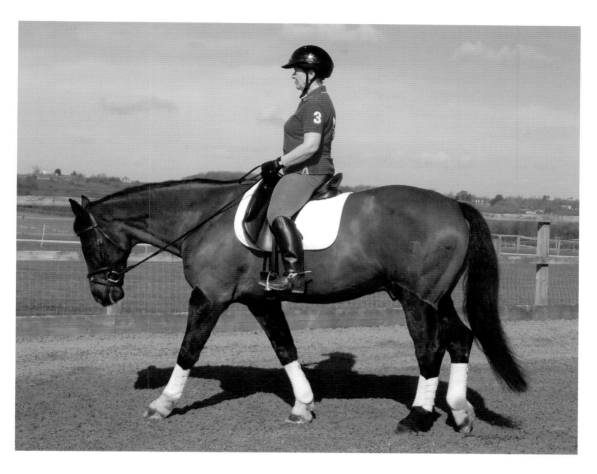

remember to do plenty of changes of gait and direction, not relying on following the outside track around the arena. Add in a few serpentines, half-circles and leg-yields to get both you and your horse thinking.

Your Seat

When warming-up your horse, or if you are about to go for a hack, allow your horse a long rein and spend a few moments getting comfortable and sit in the 'middle'; in the horse's centre of gravity. In dressage, the centre of gravity is generally further back because of the way the horse is worked, whereas in showjumping or cross-country the centre of gravity is further forward, plus the rider adapts a half-seat out of the saddle to tackle the fences. As a rider you must feel happy in these different positions and be able to adapt easily according to the dictates of the moment if you are eventing.

When riding, think of it as you bringing your mind to the partnership while your horse is bringing his four legs and his willingness to do the job – it is up to you to control these assets!

Your main aids are your seat, legs and voice. You can influence the horse to the greatest degree through your seat. You need to sit *in* – or even feel as if you are sitting *through* the saddle and feel your seat bones. Through this you can find your sense of balance – and it is this which can be improved so much through Pilates, thus achieving an independent seat.

Twenty Minute Mind-body Warm-up

The warm-up is not just for your horse – it is for you too. When next warming-up or grabbing a quick workout when you are on a tight schedule, don't think of all the things you want to achieve with your horse, such as shoulder-in, cantering on the correct leg, or focusing on the correct diagonal. How often have you come home from work in the

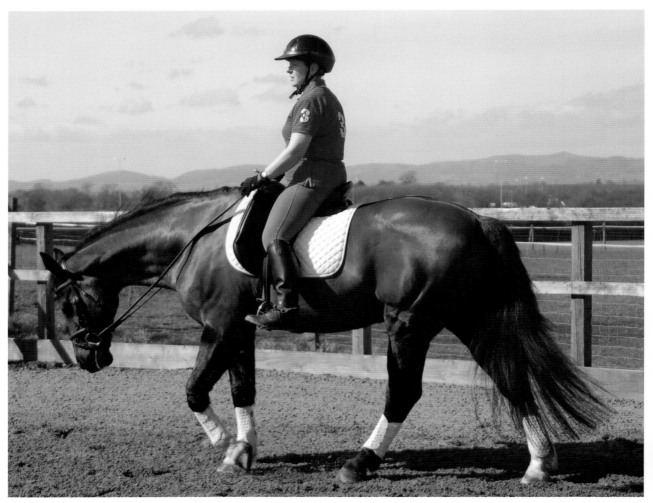

evening – or, if you are a professional rider and need to ride eight horses a day – rushed into the arena, thinking of what you need to cram in next and how you can only spend twenty minutes riding? Try instead to concentrate just on yourself – you will be amazed that once you stop trying to control your mount perfectly and relax a little and concentrate on yourself, you will find that your horse instantly goes better.

The Gaits

Once you have established where your centre of gravity is in the walk, establish it in the trot, by rising and sitting over the centre of gravity with a still body and in balance. Don't worry about where the horse's head is, just find your rhythm and, if it helps, try counting one two, one two, one two until you establish a steady trot in balance. This is a great way to warm up your body and will help you to avoid

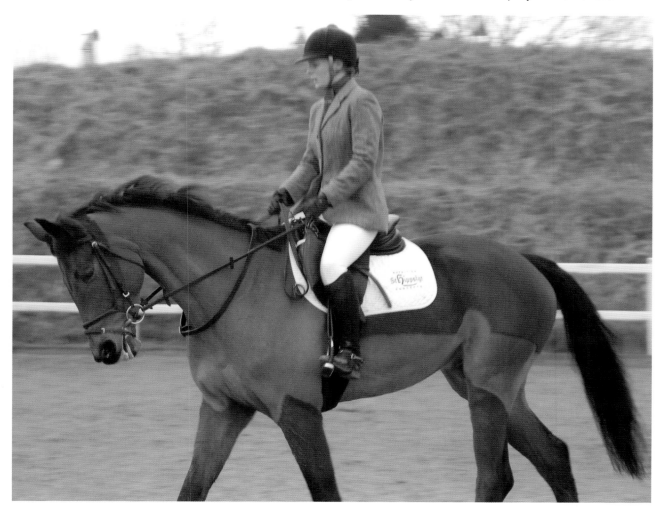

imbalances and injuries from favouring a certain rein or leg.

Once you feel in balance and relaxed in trot, move forwards into canter, concentrating on becoming soft and rhythmical through your pelvis; allowing your tailbone to curl under your body and freeing up your pelvis to move forwards and backwards and almost brush the seat. Draw up your pelvic floor a little but do not force it or brace – this will just become uncomfortable with the movement of the horse. Lift your abdominal muscles by raising your ribcage and thinking of drawing your navel through to your spine to stabilise yourself in this position – this will give you instant lift without stiffness. Think of sliding your shoulder-blades down you back and elongating your neck, stabilising your shoulder-blades without fixing.

You will notice that, as your pelvis warms up and becomes freer, you will become softer as a rider through the pelvis and you can refine the movement. (You don't want to become *too* free through the pelvis so that you become unbalanced – just enough to absorb the movement and go with the horse.) As you become softer and suppler through your seat, you will become more balanced, like a pendulum, and it won't matter what the horse does underneath you, as you will remain central in the saddle with a truly independent seat.

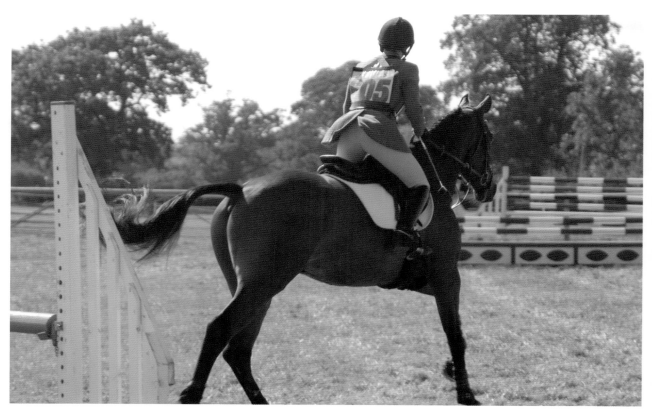

Whatever gait you are in, remember to work the horse – and thus yourself – equally on both reins.

Jumping

If you want to jump, then it is beneficial to develop a light or two-point seat, where you are slightly raised out of the saddle and balance with the aid of your core through to the balls of your feet. When adopting a light seat, you shouldn't need to tighten in the calves and thighs or – especially – hang onto the horse's mouth to balance. With good core stability work, a light seat can be achieved.

Core stability is even more important when tackling obstacles than when riding on the

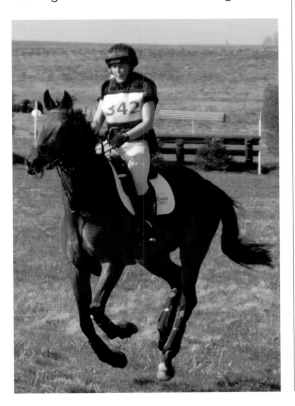

flat. You need to stay in balance when out of the saddle in your two-point seat. If you are showjumping, you need to feel comfortable doing switchbacks, curving lines, related distances and doglegs. You need to perfect your technique and energise your horse to produce the power you need for the jumping ring. When you have control over your own body, you will be able to influence your horse's stride; lengthening and shortening it as required. You will also be able to achieve the necessary calmness and stillness through your body when jumping a fence.

Likewise, if you are riding across country, you need to feel confident and balanced in your seat, which you will adapt to retain a safe and secure position as you tackle obstacles such as drops, water, steps, banks and steeplechase fences. No matter what the obstacle, it is essential that you remain over the horse's point of balance (in fact, for some fences, such as when jumping a drop or into water, for your own safety you will need to be slightly behind the movement). When galloping across country your horse's balance will be constantly challenged by the terrain and you must recognise this and adapt your seat and point of balance for maximum efficiency.

Warm-down

The warm-down is just as important for the rider as it is for the horse! Just as your horse has been working his muscles, so have you. Try to allow your horse and yourself the time to reach correct body temperature before you put him back into his stable or lorry and you yourself jump onto the next horse. Stiff muscles can often be the bane of a rider's life!

Ridden Exercises

Many of the exercises in the Pilates for Equestrians programme can be adapted to aid your fine-tuning when you are mounted. You can try these at home in the school to relax and improve your 'feel' and connection with your horse. If you have a reliable mount, you can also bring some of these exercises to the collecting ring. If not, then you can sit quietly in your trailer or lorry before your class and focus on your own body for a short time. Run through one or two of these movements to help you relax, relieve any tension and open up your upper body. And remember to breathe!

Try these!

Here are some of the exercises mentioned previously that can be adapted for use when mounted.

- Yes and No Neck Tucks and Rolls
- Shoulder Drops (with arms in front of you, lengthening out)
- Dumb Waiter
- Pelvic Tilts

- Ankle Circles
- Point and Flex
- Spine Stretch Forward
- Ribcage Closure

You can also try the exercises on the following pages

Dart Arms

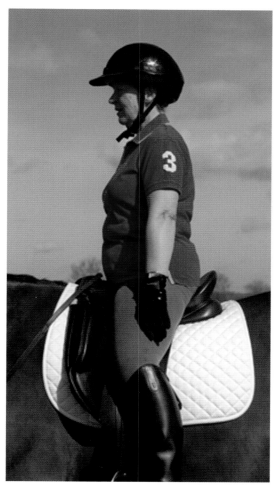

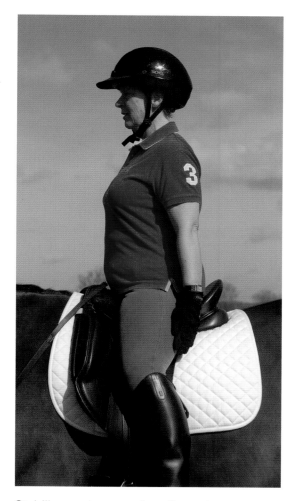

Breathe in and lengthen from the base of your spine to the crown of your head. Have your arms lengthened by your sides.

Stabilise and, as you breathe out, rotate your shoulders back in the shoulder sockets, without bracing, and gently feel your shoulder-blades relaxing down your back. Your arms will rotate at your sides, lengthening down towards your toes, palms towards your body. Breathe in to hold the position then return to the starting position.

Diamond Press Shoulders

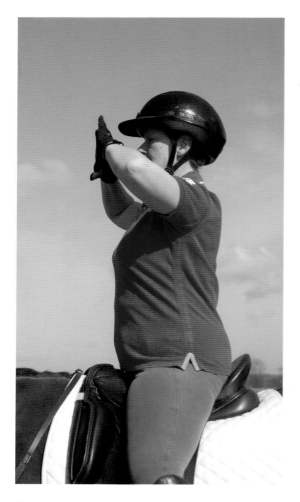

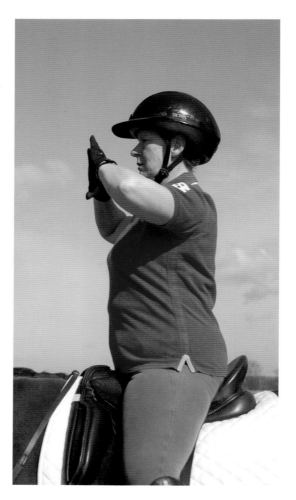

Sit tall up on your seat bones, pelvis in neutral, with your hands forming a diamond shape in front of your forehead, elbows wide. Breathe in and lengthen away from the base of your back through to the crown of your head.

Stabilise as you breathe out, lifting your chest up and forwards, opening out through the front of your collarbones, lengthening through your neck, and feel your shoulder-blades lightly gliding down your back. Breathe in to maintain the stretch, then return to the starting position.

Tree Hugging

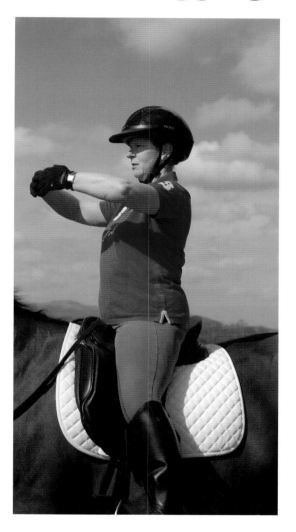 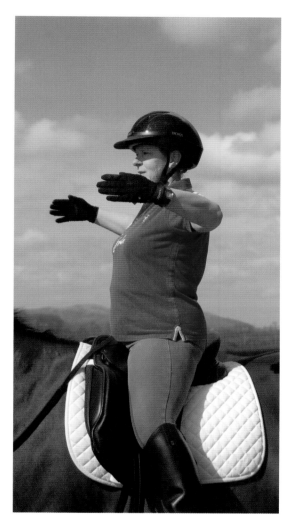

Stretch out both arms in front of you, shoulder width apart, fingertips towards each other, with elbows slightly bent as if you are hugging a tree.

Stabilise through your centre and, as you breathe in, move your arms out to your sides, keeping the elbows slightly bent, taking care not to brace your back. Then, as you breathe out, bring your fingertips back together, keeping the 'tree hugging' shape.

Leg Lifts

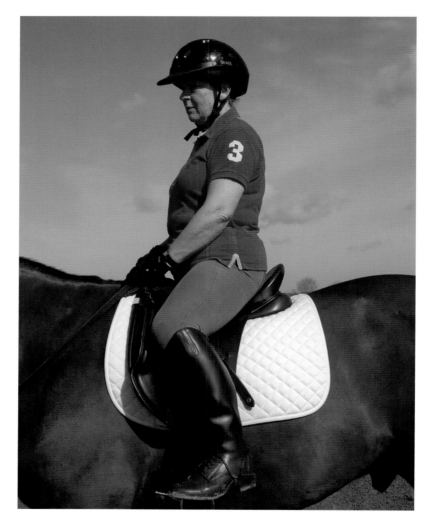

Try this simple exercise when warming-up on your horse. Drop your feet out of the stirrups, then lift your inner thighs and hips away from the saddle, in a 'D' shape with the right leg (backwards D with left leg), then drop and stretch the leg down through the thigh (which helps to lengthen your leg), open and release your hip and secure your position. Also lift your tummy, sliding your shoulder-blades down your back without bracing. Breathe wide and deep, looking straight ahead and not down.

Waist Twist

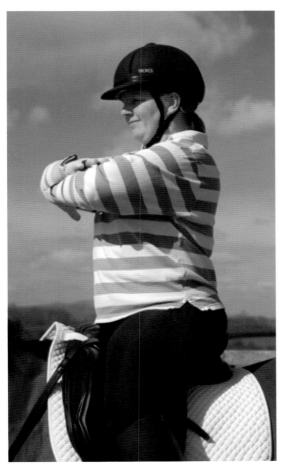

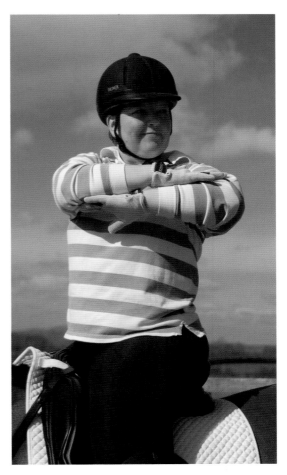

Cross your arms in front of you, ensuring that your elbows are below your shoulders (too high and it increases tension around your shoulders).

Breathe in as you lengthen your back and stretch your waist upwards, imagining the spine is a bungee then, as you breathe out, twist your upper body, head and neck around to one side. Ensure that your pelvis is squarely facing the pommel. Breathe out as your upper body comes back to the starting position, and then prepare to twist around to the opposite side.

Side Reach

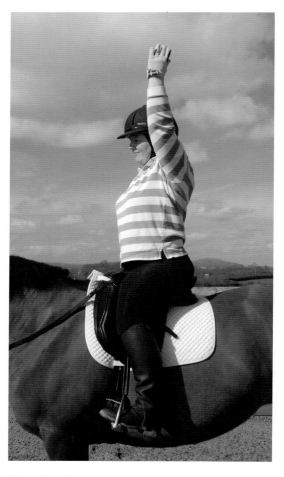 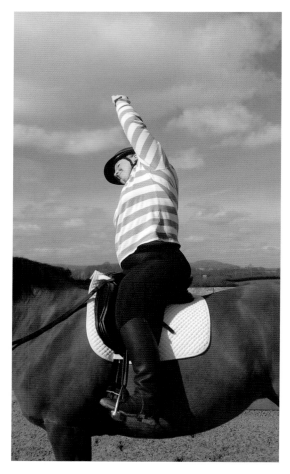

Breathe in as you lengthen your spine upwards and raise one arm up above your head, stretching your fingers up towards the sky.

Stabilise, then reach your arm up and over your head and towards the opposite side of the arena, being careful not to lean forwards or backwards. Your hips should remain still and level, not pushed out or dropping to the side. Enjoy the stretch along the side of your ribcage as you breathe in. Then return on the next out-breath and prepare to bend to the other side.

Index